Methods in Molecular Biology

Series Editor
John M. Walker
School of Life and Medical Sciences
University of Hertfordshire
Hatfield, Hertfordshire, AL10 9AB, UK

For further volumes:
http://www.springer.com/series/7651

Synthetic DNA

Methods and Protocols

Edited by

Randall A. Hughes

Applied Research Laboratories, The University of Texas at Austin, Austin, TX, USA

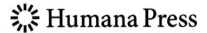 Humana Press

Editor
Randall A. Hughes
Applied Research Laboratories
The University of Texas at Austin
Austin, TX, USA

ISSN 1064-3745   ISSN 1940-6029   (electronic)
Methods in Molecular Biology
ISBN 978-1-4939-8170-0   ISBN 978-1-4939-6343-0   (eBook)
DOI 10.1007/978-1-4939-6343-0

This Humana Press imprint is published by Springer Nature
The registered company is Springer Science+Business Media LLC New York

Preface

The biological information revolution brought on by the advent of low-cost high-throughput sequencing has made available ever increasing troves of DNA sequences from all forms of life. This sequence information has provided researchers with databases of sequences which encode for all the functional (enzymes, proteins, stable RNAs) and regulatory (promoters, enhancers, ribosomal binding sites, terminators) components which make cellular biochemistry possible. These DNA sequences have served as designer templates that have enabled the recent innovations and discoveries in the fields of synthetic biology, molecular biology, biochemistry, and biological engineering. However the availability of DNA sequence information is only partly responsible for the rise in the design, study, and use of programmable engineered biological systems. Significantly, the concomitant development of tools and techniques to design, synthesize and assemble synthetic DNA into genes, synthetic circuits and even whole genomes continues to expand the applications of synthetic DNA in biology and biotechnology. This volume will present state-of-the art methods for the synthesis, design, assembly, post-synthesis processing, and application of synthetic DNA to modern biotechnology. This volume is divided into three general parts which incorporate protocols for the computational design of synthetic DNA sequences (Part I), the synthesis, assembly and cloning of synthetic DNA (Part II), and post-synthesis error reduction strategies (Part III).

The historical origins of synthetic biology methods and the production and use of synthetic DNA itself can be traced to the development of chemistries for the abiotic synthesis of DNA. In the 1970s, synthetic organic chemistry methods were developed to synthesize DNA from synthetic nucleotides. Initially these chemistries were difficult and laborious to perform but they did result in the eventual synthesis of the first functional synthetic DNA sequence which totaled 207 base pairs in length and encoded for a 75 bp tyrosine suppressor transfer RNA. Subsequent improvements to the synthetic chemistry methods in the 1980s led to the creation of the solid-phase phosphoramidite synthesis method which enabled the highly efficient, robust, and scalable synthesis of synthetic DNA. In the 1980s–1990s, recombinant DNA technologies based around the discovery and use of bacterial restriction enzyme systems and the development of the polymerase chain reaction (PCR) further contributed to the development of techniques to produce and utilize synthetic DNA. In the last decade, the growth in the interest and application of engineered biological systems and materials has led to further advancements in the design, production, processing, and use of synthetic DNA. The protocols in this volume will aid researchers who wish to produce and utilize synthetic DNA in their work and undoubtedly contribute to continued innovation in synthetic biology.

In Part I, protocols which outline the use of three computational tools for the design of synthetic oligonucleotide sequences for a variety of applications are outlined. In Chapter 1, Damien O'Halloran provides a guide for the use of the online STITCHER algorithm for designing DNA sequences for overlap assembly. This program would be useful for those desiring to assemble longer DNA sequences from shorter starting materials by PCR assembly based methods for a variety of applications including gene synthesis and synthetic pathway construction. In Chapter 2, Yu et al. present the online codon optimization tool called "COOL." This protocol allows researchers to use the COOL program to recode and codon optimize synthetic DNA sequences to reflect the codon preferences of a host organism or user defined codon tables. This tool would be especially useful for those that wish to optimize a synthetic gene for increased expression in a heterologous host organism. Codon shuffling of a DNA sequence could also be used to tweak the expression of genes in a biosynthetic pathway to optimize metabolic flux through a multigene system. In Chapter 3, Milligan and Garry present the use of the Shuffle Optimizer program for recoding homologous genes for synthesis and subsequent molecular shuffling. This algorithm would be very useful for researchers who are interesting in the directed evolution of proteins via in vitro shuffling methods as it allows for maximizing the potential cross-overs during the shuffling protocol. Recoding homologs to more closely match host codon preferences and maximizing sequence homology between genes would enhance the creation of libraries for directed evolution and allow researchers to explore greater sequence diversity by directed evolution.

Beyond the (re-)design of DNA sequences for assembly, expression, and evolution the assembly of DNA sequences from smaller pieces into larger genes, pathways, or constructs is important for the engineering of encoded biological function. This volume contains a series of protocols which allow the researcher to assemble and/or clone DNA of various sizes into larger constructs for subsequent testing and application. One popular application of synthetic DNA is for the directed evolution of biomolecular function. Directed evolution is a powerful tool that can be used to augment the substrate specificity of enzymes and binding proteins as well as improve the stability and function of proteins and other biomolecules. In all directed evolution techniques a library of nucleic acid (DNA, RNA) variants is created and parsed by a functional screen or selection to select for a desired function. Efficient library construction and cloning is essential to successfully perform direct evolution experiments. To this end, in Chapter 4 Zhong et al. present a protocol for overlap PCR-based cloning and preparation of random mutagenesis libraries for evolution in *E. coli*. This protocol provides an efficient method for generating libraries of protein variants and cloning them using a straightforward PCR-based method. In Chapter 5, Currin et al. present the "SpeedyGenes" method for assembling synthetic genes from single-stranded oligonucleotides. This method allows for the accurate assembly and cloning of genes and gene variant libraries directly from oligonucleotides. A similar method detailed in Chapter 10 entitled polymerase step reaction (PSR) developed by Brian DeDecker can be used to create genes or gene libraries from oligonucleotides without PCR in a simple and accurate protocol which has been successfully used to synthesize phage display libraries. These protocols add useful techniques to the molecular toolbox of experimenters using directed evolution techniques to augment biological function.

In addition to directed evolution applications, several other protocols in this volume will aid researchers in the hierarchical assembly of DNA constructs for utilization in a number of other synthetic biology applications. In Chapter 6, Storch et al. introduce a modular assembly method they call BASIC. This method uses DNA linkers to mediate the assembly of modular DNA assemblies into larger constructs guided by designed prefix and suffix sequences. This method allows for the flexible and accurate assembly of modular DNA constructs into complete expression constructs, biosynthetic pathways, or combinatorial sequence libraries. The authors have demonstrated >90 % assembly accuracy for constructs containing up to seven component DNA parts. Similarly, the PaperClip assembly method presented in Chapter 9 allows for the assembly of multiple DNA parts using short "clip" adapter sequences in a simple and flexible protocol. Both of these methods are attractive alternatives to the BioBrick and similar assembly standards commonly used in synthetic biology applications and provide a level of accuracy and flexibility which is superior to these traditional standards. Additional assembly methods in Chapters 8 and 12 present methods to allow researchers to assemble DNA sequences from single-stranded DNA oligonucleotides by the highly accurate ligase cycling reaction (Chapter 8) and to assemble DNA constructs using the robust and highly efficient GoldenGATEway method (Chapter 12). Assembly and manipulation of DNA in vivo by taking advantage of the native yeast homologous recombination system has become a powerful tool for the assembly of DNA constructs especially those that are multi-kilobases or greater in length. To these ends, protocols in Chapters 13 and 14 allow researchers to use yeast to manipulate DNA sequences for genetic manipulation by gene deletion (Chapter 13) and the hierarchical assembly of DNA constructs from smaller pieces of DNA (Chapter 14).

The use of synthetic DNA for manipulating genomic DNA or mobile genetic elements such as expression vectors is a hallmark of many molecular biology experiments. Therefore methods which reduce the complexity, labor, time, and expense associated with these techniques would be of great utility to researchers in the molecular biosciences. In Chapter 11, Cui and Sherwin present the Clonetegration method for assembling DNA and integrating it into bacterial genomes. This method uses bacteriophage integrases to facilitate the cloning, assembly, and integration of DNA into bacterial chromosomes. This method provides a simple and rapid strategy to manipulate bacterial genomic DNA and should prove useful to both academic and industrial scientists interested in bacterial genomic manipulation and strain creation. In Chapters 15 and 16 methods are presented which allow researchers to construct and manipulate plasmid DNA sequences for a variety of applications. Krishnamurthy and Zhang present a method for the rapid manipulation of plasmid DNA templates (Chapter 15) by simultaneous deletion and reassembly by PCR which will allow researchers to tailor existing vector sequences to their particular application. In Chapter 16, Jajesniak and Wong introduce the Quickstep-Cloning method for construction of recombinant plasmids which provides a convenient method for assembling expression constructs and synthetic biological circuits.

To round out this volume, methods which address sequence errors inherent in chemically synthesized DNA are presented. Sequence errors are introduced into synthetic DNA due to reaction inefficiencies during the oligonucleotide synthesis process as well as by DNA polymerases during the assembly of dsDNA during the assembly process. To ensure sequence fidelity, enrichment of correct sequences from raw synthetic DNA populations which have sequences that both contain and lack errors is an important part of processing and using synthetic DNA. Applications which require ssDNA oligonucleotides with very high sequence fidelity may require expensive post-synthesis purification or treatment of chemically synthesized ssDNA oligonucleotides before use. One alternative to chemically synthesized ssDNA oligonucleotides is to utilize DNA produced biologically which generally contain fewer errors. To this end, in Chapter 7 Ducani and Hogberg present a method for the enzymatic synthesis of ssDNA oligonucleotides for applications where high fidelity oligonucleotides are required. In the last few years the use of multiplex microarray synthesized oligonucleotide pools for gene synthesis has emerged as a low-cost alternative to traditional column synthesized oligonucleotides. However the synthesis fidelity of microarray synthesized oligonucleotides is generally lower than that of the traditional column synthesized oligonucleotides. In Chapter 17 Wan et al. present a MutS-mediated method to enrich for oligonucleotides and assembled dsDNAs without errors from microarray synthesized oligonucleotide pools. This protocol provides researchers with a straightforward and inexpensive method to utilize oligonucleotide pools as starting materials for gene synthesis while eliminating the associated sequence errors.

For DNA sequences assembled from oligonucleotides which contain a protein encoding sequence (or at least lack a termination codon), a simple and useful method for eliminating the majority of the errors is to fuse the synthetic coding sequence to a reporter gene and then screen for functional reporters by an in vivo phenotype screen. This type of screen works based on the necessity to maintain the correct reading frame of the fused reporter gene during translation to express a functional reporter protein. Since most synthesis-related errors are single or double nucleotide deletions, sequences which contain one of these deletion mutations will cause a shift in the translational reading frame which will result in the failed expression of the fused reporter protein. In Chapter 18, Hoshida et al. outline the use of such a system in yeast for the selection of error-free synthetic genes from raw synthesis products. This method will be of use for any researcher synthesizing protein encoding genes and needs to enrich for correct sequences from synthetic products. In addition, since this reading frame selection is designed to work in yeast, researchers can take advantage of the power of the yeast recombination system to enable cloning and in vivo assembly of their synthetic DNA constructs prior to error selection.

This book should be of use to researchers in the molecular biosciences who need to manipulate DNA sequences in the course of their work. The protocols and methods outlined herein contain innovative methods for the design, synthesis, assembly, cloning, and screening of synthetic DNA sequences which will help researchers advance the understanding of basic biology as well as the manipulation of biological systems for a variety of applications. I wish to thank all of the contributors to this volume for sharing their expertise and their methods with the research community. Finally, I want to thank my colleagues at the University of Texas-Applied Research Laboratories for their generous encouragement and support in the advancement of basic and applied science and engineering in the biological sciences and beyond.

Austin, TX, USA   *Randall A. Hughes*

Contents

PART I   COMPUTATIONAL TOOLS FOR DESIGN AND ASSEMBLY
              OF SYNTHETIC DNA

PART II   DNA SYNTHESIS, ASSEMBLY, AND CLONING

Contributors

RINJI AKADA • *Department of Applied Chemistry, Graduate School of Science and Technology for Innovation, Yamaguchi University, Ube, Japan; Research Center for Thermotolerant Microbial Resources, Yamaguchi University, Yamaguchi, Japan; Yamaguchi University Biomedical Engineering Center, Ube, Japan*

KOK SIONG ANG • *Department of Chemical and Biomolecular Engineering, National University of Singapore, Singapore*

GEOFF S. BALDWIN • *Department of Life Sciences, Centre for Synthetic Biology and Innovation, Imperial College London, London, UK*

ARTURO CASINI • *Department of Life Sciences, Centre for Synthetic Biology and Innovation, Imperial College London, London, UK*

SUNIL CHANDRAN • *Amyris, Inc., Emeryville, CA, USA*

LUN CUI • *Synthetic Biology Group, Institute Pasteur, Paris, France*

ANDREW CURRIN • *Manchester Institute of Biotechnology, The University of Manchester, Manchester, UK; School of Chemistry, The University of Manchester, Manchester, UK; Centre for Synthetic Biology of Fine and Speciality Chemicals (SYNBIOCHEM), The University of Manchester, Manchester, UK*

PHILIP J. DAY • *Manchester Institute of Biotechnology, The University of Manchester, Manchester, UK; Centre for Synthetic Biology of Fine and Speciality Chemicals (SYNBIOCHEM), The University of Manchester, Manchester, UK; Faculty of Medical and Human Sciences, The University of Manchester, Manchester, UK*

BRIAN S. DEDECKER • *Department of Molecular, Cellular and Developmental Biology, University of Colorado, Boulder, CO, USA*

COSIMO DUCANI • *Department of Medical Biochemistry and Biophysics, Karolinska Institutet, Stockholm, Sweden*

ALISTAIR ELFICK • *School of Engineering, University of Edinburgh, Edinburgh, UK*

TOM ELLIS • *Department of Bioengineering, Centre for Synthetic Biology and Innovation, Imperial College London, London, UK*

CHRISTOPHER E. FRENCH • *School of Biological Sciences, University of Edinburgh, Edinburgh, UK*

XIAOLIAN GAO • *School of Life Science, University of Science and Technology of China, Hefei, Anhui, Republic of China; Hefei National Laboratory for Physical Science at the Microscale, Hefei, Anhui, People's Republic China*

DANIEL J. GARRY • *The Department of Molecular Biosciences, The University of Texas at Austin, Austin, TX, USA*

KWANG-LAE HOE • *Department of New Drug Discovery and Development, Chungnam National University, Daejeon, South Korea*

BJÖRN HÖGBERG • *Department of Medical Biochemistry and Biophysics, Karolinska Institutet, Stockholm, Sweden*

JIONG HONG • *School of Life Science, University of Science and Technology of China, Hefei, Anhui, Republic of China; Hefei National Laboratory for Physical Science at the Microscale, Hefei, Anhui, People's Republic China*

HISASHI HOSHIDA • *Department of Applied Chemistry, Graduate School of Science and Technology for Innovation, Yamaguchi University, Ube, Japan; Research Center for Thermotolerant Microbial Resources, Yamaguchi University, Yamaguchi, Japan; Yamaguchi University Biomedical Engineering Center, Ube, Japan*

PAWEL JAJESNIAK • *ChELSI Institute and Advanced Biomanufacturing Centre, Department of Chemical and Biological Engineering, University of Sheffield, Sheffield, UK*

DOUGLAS B. KELL • *Manchester Institute of Biotechnology, The University of Manchester, Manchester, UK; School of Chemistry, The University of Manchester, Manchester, UK; Centre for Synthetic Biology of Fine and Speciality Chemicals (SYNBIOCHEM), The University of Manchester, Manchester, UK*

DONG-UK KIM • *Aging Research Center, Korea Research Institute of Bioscience and Biotechnology (KRIBB), Daejeon, South Korea*

JINSIL KIM • *Aging Research Center, Korea Research Institute of Bioscience and Biotechnology (KRIBB), Daejeon, South Korea*

STEPHAN KIRCHMAIER • *COS – Centre for Organismal Studies, Heidelberg University, Heidelberg, Germany*

VISHNU KRISHNAMURTHY • *Department of Biochemistry, School of Molecular and Cellular Biology, University of Illinois at Urbana-Champaign, Urbana, IL, USA*

DONG-YUP LEE • *Department of Chemical and Biomolecular Engineering, National University of Singapore, Singapore, Singapore; NUS Synthetic Biology for Clinical and Technological Innovation (SynCTI), Life Sciences Institute, National University of Singapore, Singapore, Singapore; Bioprocessing Technology Institute, Agency for Science, Technology and Research (A*STAR), Singapore, Singapore*

CHAO-KUO LIU • *School of Biological Sciences, University of Edinburgh, Edinburgh, UK*

KATHARINA LUST • *COS – Centre for Organismal Studies, Heidelberg University, Heidelberg, Germany*

BEN MACKROW • *Department of Life Sciences, Centre for Synthetic Biology and Innovation, Imperial College London, London, UK*

JOHN N. MILLIGAN • *The Department of Molecular Biosciences, The University of Texas at Austin, Austin, TX, USA*

DAMIEN M. O'HALLORAN • *Department of Biology and Institute for Neuroscience, The George Washington University, Washington, DC, USA*

ALEJANDRO SALINAS • *School of Biological Sciences, University of Edinburgh, Edinburgh, UK*

ELAINE SHAPLAND • *Amyris, Inc., Emeryville, CA, USA*

KEITH E. SHEARWIN • *Department of Molecular and Cellular Biology, School of Biological Science, University of Adelaide, Adelaide, SA, Australia*

MARKO STORCH • *Department of Life Sciences, Centre for Synthetic Biology and Innovation, Imperial College London, London, UK*

NEIL SWAINSTON • *Manchester Institute of Biotechnology, The University of Manchester, Manchester, UK; Centre for Synthetic Biology of Fine and Speciality Chemicals (SYNBIOCHEM), The University of Manchester, Manchester, UK; School of Computer Science, The University of Manchester, Manchester, UK*

MARYIA TRUBITSYNA • *School of Biological Sciences, University of Edinburgh, Edinburgh, UK*

WEN WAN • *School of Life Science, University of Science and Technology of China, Hefei, Anhui, People's Republic China*

DONGMEI WANG • *School of Life Science, University of Science and Technology of China, Hefei, Anhui, People's Republic China*

PING WEI • *College of Biotechnology and Pharmaceutical Engineering, Nanjing Tech University, Nanjing, China*

JOCHEN WITTBRODT • *COS – Centre for Organismal Studies, Heidelberg University, Heidelberg, Germany*

TUCK SENG WONG • *ChELSI Institute and Advanced Biomanufacturing Centre, Department of Chemical and Biological Engineering, University of Sheffield, Sheffield, UK*

TOHRU YARIMIZU • *Department of Applied Chemistry, Graduate School of Science and Technology for Innovation, Yamaguchi University, Ube, Japan*

CHUN YOU • *Biological Systems Engineering Department, Virginia Tech, Blacksburg, VA, USA; Cell Free Bioinnovations Inc., Blacksburg, VA, USA; Tianjin Institute of Industrial Biotechnology, Chinese Academy of Sciences, Tianjin, China*

KAI YU • *Department of Chemical and Biomolecular Engineering, National University of Singapore, Singapore, Singapore; NUS Synthetic Biology for Clinical and Technological Innovation (SynCTI), Life Sciences Institute, National University of Singapore, Singapore, Singapore*

KAI ZHANG • *Department of Biochemistry, School of Molecular and Cellular Biology, University of Illinois at Urbana-Champaign, Urbana, IL, USA*

YI-HENG PERCIVAL ZHANG • *Biological Systems Engineering Department, Virginia Tech, Blacksburg, VA, USA; Cell Free Bioinnovations Inc., Blacksburg, VA, USA; Tianjin Institute of Industrial Biotechnology, Chinese Academy of Sciences, Tianjin, China*

CHAO ZHONG • *Biological Systems Engineering Department, Virginia Tech, Blacksburg, VA, USA; College of Biotechnology and Pharmaceutical Engineering, Nanjing Tech University, Nanjing, China*

Part I

Computational Tools for Design and Assembly of Synthetic DNA

Chapter 1

A Guide to Using *STITCHER* for Overlapping Assembly PCR Applications

Damien M. O'Halloran

Abstract

Overlapping PCR is commonly used in many molecular applications that include stitching PCR fragments together, generating fluorescent transcriptional and translational fusions, inserting mutations, making deletions, and PCR cloning. Overlapping PCR is also used for genotyping and in detection experiments using techniques such as loop-mediated isothermal amplification (LAMP). STITCHER is a web tool providing a central resource for researchers conducting all types of overlapping assembly PCR experiments with an intuitive interface for automated primer design that's fast, easy to use, and freely available online.

Key words PCR, Overlapping PCR, Assembly PCR, Primer design, PCR fusion, Molecular biology

---

1 Introduction

Overlapping PCR can be used for a wide number of experiments, including "stitching" PCR fragments together, generating GFP/RFP transcriptional and translational fusions, inserting mutations, making deletion mutations, and *L*oop-mediated isothermal *AMP*ification (LAMP) [1–5]. STITCHER is a web-based tool (Fig. 1), which aims to provide researchers conducting all types of overlapping PCR applications with a fast, easy to use, automated method for returning all necessary primers [6]. STITCHER can handle both single sequence input and multisequence input. STITCHER can be used to provide primers for removing sections of DNA using the "deletion mutation" feature or inserting mutations using the "user-defined overlapping sequence" feature. STITCHER can also search for off-target sites for selected primers on each strand for specific species.

Randall A. Hughes (ed.), *Synthetic DNA: Methods and Protocols*, Methods in Molecular Biology, vol. 1472,
DOI 10.1007/978-1-4939-6343-0_1, © Springer Science+Business Media New York 2017

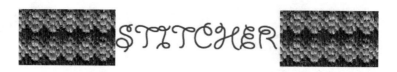

stitcher | fetch | off-target | blast-off | cross-comp | articles | help

STITCHER: a web resource for high-throughput design of primers for overlapping PCR applications

Enter any number of sequences in FASTA format:

```
>sample fastA format
ATGACCAAGTTGAAAATCTACTTGTTCCTTGTTGTCTCGTTGACTACACTTGGGCAAT
ACGCAGCTGAGCCGCAAAATGGAGAAATAATTCACGTATCTTCCCAACGTATACCCG
GGCCTGAGCCGGCTTGTGCTCCGGCTAAGCCATGTTCCCCCGGAGTTATCGTACCA
GTTTGGCAGCCATCGGAAAACCTGTCAGAATGCAAAATATGGTTCCGTGCAATTGTC
TATTTAATCGCATTGGCCTATTTATTCTTTGGTGTCTCAATTGTGGCGGATCGATTCA
TGGCGTCTATTGAAGTGATCACTTCTCAGCAGAAATCTGTGAAAATGAAGAAGATAA
CCGGTGAACATTTCACAATAATGGTACGTGTCTGGAATGAAACAGTCAGTAACCTGA
CGCTAATGGCTCTCGGATCCTCAGCCCCCGAGATTTTGCTCTCGGTCATTGAAATTT
GCGGAAATAATTTCGAAGCTGGAGAGCTGGGACCATCGACAATTGTTGGATCAGCTG
```

Primer size:
Max: 28   Min: 18

5' and 3' search areas (bp):
5': 100   3': 100

Primer GC %:
Upper GC: 60   Lower GC: 40

Primer Tm:
Upper Tm: 68   Lower Tm: 55

Salt concentration (mM):
○ 10 ● 50

Increment forward:
Steps (bps): 2

Increment reverse:
Steps (bps): 2

GC clamp:
○ Yes ● No

Self complementarity stringency:
● Regular ○ High ○ None

Exclude repetitive sequence:
● Yes ○ No

Overlapping fragment:
none

User-defined overlapping reverse sequence:

User-defined overlapping forward sequence:

Deletion Mutation:
○ Yes ● No

Fig. 1 Screenshot from the STITCHER home page. Default settings are inserted for all parameters and also a sample sequence is provided in FASTA format. The navigation menu at the top of the page can be used to obtain sequences from NCBI (fetch), search for off-target matches (off-target and blast-off), examine cross complementary between primers (cross-comp), read about overlapping PCR technology (articles), and learn more about STITCHER's features and output (help)

2 Materials

STITCHER can be found on the Internet at http://ohalloranlab.
net/STITCHER.html (Fig. 1). STITCHER was written using
Perl, CSS, JavaScript, and HTML. STITCHER has been tested on
PC and MAC, as well as iPhone and Android mobile devices, using
the following browsers: Safari, Chrome, Internet Explorer, Firefox,
and Atomic. If STITCHER does not recognize your browser, it will
return a warning. STITCHER is free to use without login require-
ments, and therefore the end user only needs a computer with
Internet connectivity and one of the browsers listed above to use it.

3 Methods

3.1 STITCHER Parameters

3.1.1 Input

1. All input sequences for STITCHER must be in FASTA format
   [7]. FASTA format starts with a ">" character followed by a
   definition, all on the same line. STITCHER is not case sensitive,
   and the DNA sequence begins on the next line for example:

   > gene_1 name
   ATGGTAGTATCAGCTAGCATCAGTTAG

2. The upper and lower range for primer size is provided as whole
   integers (*see* **Note 1**).

3.1.2 Search Area

1. STITCHER only searches for primers within the user specified
   5′ and 3′ search areas (Fig. 2).

2. STITCHER will loop over the specified search area and return
   primers that match all other criteria that sit in the primer length
   range such that lower length ≤ primer ≤ upper length.

3. A user setting the 5′ search to 200 bps will result in STITCHER
   searching for primers within the first 200 bps. If the 5′ or 3′
   search areas are greater than the size of the input DNA
   sequence, this will result in a failed program execution. The 5′
   and 3′ search area can be of different sizes, and including this
   feature allows the user to determine the product range, which
   is also returned in the output HTML file.

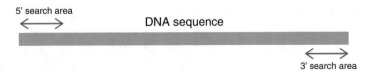

Fig. 2 STITCHER only searches for primers within the user designated 5′ and 3′
search areas. The *blue line* indicates the DNA sequence

4. If the user selects "Deletion Mutation," the 5′ and 3′ search areas become the fixed nucleotide number for the deletion area. Following the example above where the user sets the 5′ and 3′ search areas to 200 bps; if the user also selects "deletion mutation," STITCHER will only return one primer pair starting at 200 bps in the case of the forward primer that contains a reverse complement overlap to the reverse primer overlap, and starting at 200 bps before the end of the input sequence the reverse primer will be generated, assuming that all the selected criteria can be met.

3.1.3   Primer GC% and T_m Calculation

1. Forward and reverse primer pairs should have similar T_m values and similar GC% values. The GC% is calculated by STITCHER by counting the number of G and C nucleotides and dividing by the total number of nucleotides (A, C, G, T) and multiplying this number by 100 to get a percentage.

2. Undetermined base pairs can be included using the letter "N". In the case of the reverse primer that contains either a pre-defined overlap (e.g., GFP or mCherry) or a user-defined overlap: the GC% is calculated only from the designed portion (i.e., not the overlap—this is also the case for primer T_m values) (*see* **Notes 2** and **3**).

3. The default formula used to calculate the primer melting temperature (T_m) assumes that the reaction is carried out in the presence of 50 mM monovalent cations (this can be changed to reflect reactions at 10 mM) using the nearest neighbor thermodynamic calculations as follows for primers less than 36 bases:

$$Tm = \Delta H / (\Delta S + R \times ln(c/4)) - 273.15 + 16.6 \, log[K^+]$$

where ΔH (enthalpic) and ΔS (entropic) are as described in [8, 9] and R is the molar gas constant, and c is the total molar concentration of the annealing oligonucleotides when not self-complementary. For primers greater than 36 bases the following formula is used:

$$T_m = 81.5\,°C + 16.6\,°C \, x \left(log10[Na^+] + [K^+]\right) + 0.41\,°C \, x \, (\%GC) \quad 675/N$$

where N is primer length.

3.1.4   Increments Along the Search Area

1. STITCHER moves along the input DNA in set increments (bps) determined by the user. The default step is 2 bps. Lowering the step increment increases the number of primers returned. However, in several instances (e.g., Primer walking or LAMP), defined increments are preferred to return possible primer sequences. Therefore, the increment step can be set by the user by entering the number representing nucleotide counts along the input sequence.

3.1.5 Self-Complementarity and Repetitive Sequence

1. Intramolecular primer interactions can occur if the primer exhibits excessive self-complementarity. The level of excess is determined by setting a stringency control to "Regular" (default), "High," or "None."

2. STITCHER can calculate three self-complementarity scores: one score for the forward primer; one score for the designed reverse primer; and one score for the designed reverse primer/overlap chimera. Determining the "Regular" stringency score was done in silico by examining the number of primers returned from random input sequences, and also experimentally by testing returned primers of "regular" stringency scores to ensure robust PCR products were generated. The "High" stringency score will significantly reduce the number of primers returned (*see* **Note 4**).

3. STITCHER's default mode is to exclude repetitive sequence, and in doing so STITCHER will void primer sequences that contain >4 identical base pairs, e.g., "AAAAA" or "GGGGG" (4 bp homopolymeric repeats are okay).

4. By excluding repetitive sequence, STITCHER will also select against any sequence that contains four or more dinucleotide repeats (e.g., ATATATAT or GCGCGCGC). These repetitive sequences will significantly increase intramolecular interactions; however, in the case of repetitive sequence inputs this feature can be de-selected.

3.1.6 Overlap Fragment

1. Using the drop-down selection feature the user can select a predefined overlapping fragment (Fig. 3). Currently these include sequences for:

GFP: ACAGCTCCTCGCCCTTGCTCACCAT

mCherry: TATCTTCTTCACCCTTTGAGACCAT

RFP: TATCTTCTTCACCCTTTGAGACCAT

YFP: ACAGCTCCTCGCCCTTGCTCACCAT

tdTomato: TGACCTCCTCGCCCTTGCTCACCAT

GFP_C_elegans: AGTCGACCTGCAGGCATGCAAGCT

Illumina Paired End Adapter1:ACACTCTTTCCCTACAC GACGCTCTTCCGATCT

Illumin Paired End Adapter 2CTCGGCATTCCTGCTGAAC CGCTCTTCCGATCT

Illumina Paired End PCR Primer 1:AATGATACGGCGACCAC CGAGATCTACACTCTTTCCCTACACGACGCT CTTCCGATCT

Illumina Paired End PCR Primer 2: CAAGCAGAAGACG GCATACGAGATCGGTCTCGGCATTCCTGCT GAACCGCTCTTCCGATCT

Illumina Paired End Sequencing Primer 1:

ACACTCTTTCCCTACACGACGCTCTTCCGATCT

Illumina Paired End Sequencing Primer 2:

CGGTCTCGGCATTCCTACTGAACCGCTCTTCC
GATCT

2. The overlap sequences can be used to generate transcriptional or translational reporters fused to various fluorophores; it can also be used in Illumina paired end sequencing reactions. In the case of "GFP_Celegans," the sequence is a commonly used overlap to stitch "GFP" to a gene or promoter of interest (see [5, 10] for more details) (*see* **Note 5**).

3. As per the "user-defined reverse overlap" textbox, the "user-defined forward overlap" textbox can be used to add any sequence to the 5′ end of the forward primer. In most cases, users will want to design primers with a specific overlap to their input DNA. In these cases, the user can input a DNA sequence in the "forward" or "reverse" (or both) overlap sequence textboxes and the primers that are returned will contain the user specified overlap sequence of any length.

3.1.7 Deletion Overlap

1. Overlapping PCR can be used to delete segments of DNA (Fig. 3). In this case the user will usually have a specific area in mind to be deleted and therefore using 5′ and 3′ search areas will not make sense. If the user selects the "deletion mutation" feature the values entered in the 5′ and 3′ search area text boxes will be used to generate a single primer pair that starts from the base pair entered in the 5′ and 3′ search area text boxes.

2. By selecting the "deletion mutation" feature the forward primer will automatically contain a reverse complement match at its 5′ end to the reverse primer's overlapping segment; thus, the user only needs to enter a sequence for the "reverse overlap" and not the "forward overlap."

3.2 Remotely Retrieving Sequences

STITCHER also includes a tool called "fetch" that will return sequences from NCBI using Entrez Programming Utilities [www.ncbi.nlm.nih.gov/books/NBK25501/]. To use fetch, the user inputs one or more accession numbers into the textbox, and after clicking "submit," the program returns the nucleotide sequences in FASTA format by printing to the browser.

3.3 Off-Target Detection

1. Once a primer of interest is selected using the features outlined above, it can then be screened for off-target hits using STITCHER's "off-target detection" feature (*see* **Note 6**).

2. The user can enter the number of mismatches permitted in the off-target search. An integer must be entered in this box. Use zero for no mismatches. Also, if this feature is selected STITCHER can examine both strands of DNA for potential

Data input & application	Representative Overview	STITCHER features
Primer design for multiple DNA input sequences	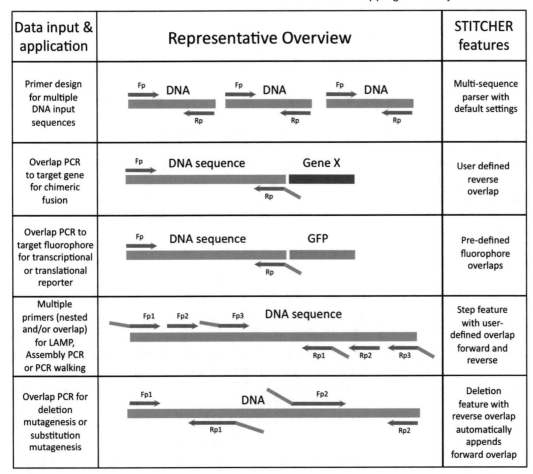	Multi-sequence parser with default settings
Overlap PCR to target gene for chimeric fusion		User defined reverse overlap
Overlap PCR to target fluorophore for transcriptional or translational reporter		Pre-defined fluorophore overlaps
Multiple primers (nested and/or overlap) for LAMP, Assembly PCR or PCR walking		Step feature with user-defined overlap forward and reverse
Overlap PCR for deletion mutagenesis or substitution mutagenesis		Deletion feature with reverse overlap automatically appends forward overlap

Fig. 3 Overview of the main STITCHER facilitated PCR applications. In the *left column* the cartoon indicates input type and the desired applications, which are then represented in cartoon form in the *middle column*. The *column on the right* indicates the STITCHER specific features that enable each application

off-target matches incorporating in each case the number of mismatches entered in the mismatch textbox.

3.4 Remote BLAST Searches

The user can remotely perform BLAST searches using the "blast-off" tool to search for off-target hits against NCBI's nucleotide non-redundant database. Output from the BLAST search is printed to the browser. This facility can be useful to search for nonspecific primer matches.

3.5 Checking Cross Complementarity

The cross complementarity tool allows the user to input forward and reverse primers, and calculates the free energy ($\Delta G°$kj/mol) of DNA duplexes using the formula:

$$\Delta G° \left(total \right) = \Delta H°_{total} - T \Delta S°_{total}$$

where enthalpic, ΔH°, and entropic, ΔS°, parameters are as described in [11]. The cross complementarity tool also returns a warning if significant complementarity exists between each primer, where significance was tuned based upon Primer3Plus [12] complementarity values from 100 primer pairs. Users can input the selected primer pairs and test for significant primer dimer using STITCHER's cross complementarity tool.

3.6 Literature Search on Overlapping PCR Applications

The end user can also stay up to date with recent articles related to overlapping PCR technology through STITCHER's "articles" page. Clicking "get papers" or "get more papers" will return matches for articles related to overlapping PCR.

4 Notes

1. Usually, primer lengths from 18 base pairs to 28 bps work well for routine PCR conditions.

2. The presence of a GC dinucleotide combination at the 3′ end of the primer facilitates specific binding on account of the greater strength in bonds between G and C base pairs. If this feature is selected, STITCHER will only return primers where a suitable GC dinucleotide combination at the 3′ end of the forward primer can be detected.

3. Usually, a GC content between 40 and 60 % is appropriate.

4. Setting the score to "None" can be very useful where highly repetitive sequence is examined.

5. The user can also select none of the predefined overlapping fragments, and instead primers without overlaps can be generated for the ligation PCR step, or for traditional PCR. If the user does not want to use one of the predefined reverse overlap fragments, it is also possible to input any sequence into the "user-defined overlapping sequence" textbox and instead this sequence will be incorporated into the program.

6. As of now this function only permits screening against the following genomes:

   Tannerella_forsythia ATCC_43037_uid83157/NC_016610

   Staphylococcus_aureus_MRSA252 uid57839/NC_002952

   Candidatus_Liberibacter americanus_Sao_Paulo_ uid227424/NC_022793

   Bacillus anthracis CDC_684_uid59303/NC_012577

   Bordetella pertussis CS_uid158859/NC_017223

   Plasmodium falciparum 3D7 version 2.1.5

   Streptococcus pneumoniae ATCC_700669

Mycobacterium tuberculosis Erdman_ATCC_35801
Escherichia_coli K12_substr_W3110_uid161931
Klebsiella_pneumoniae 1084_uid174151/NC_018522

Acknowledgements

Support for this work was provided by The George Washington University (GWU) Columbian College of Arts and Sciences, GWU Office of the Vice President for Research, and the GWU Department of Biological Sciences.

References

1. Bryksin AV, Matsumura I (2010) Overlap extension PCR cloning: a simple and reliable way to create recombinant plasmids. Biotechniques 48(6):463–465. doi:10.2144/000113418

2. Heckman KL, Pease LR (2007) Gene splicing and mutagenesis by PCR-driven overlap extension. Nat Protoc 2(4):924–932, nprot.2007.132 [pii]

3. Notomi T, Okayama H, Masubuchi H et al (2000) Loop-mediated isothermal amplification of DNA. Nucleic Acids Res 28(12):E63

4. Yoshida A, Nagashima S, Ansai T et al (2005) Loop-mediated isothermal amplification method for rapid detection of the periodontopathic bacteria *Porphyromonas gingivalis*, *Tannerella forsythia*, and *Treponema denticola*. J Clin Microbiol 43(5):2418–2424, 43/5/2418 [pii]

5. Hobert O (2002) PCR fusion-based approach to create reporter gene constructs for expression analysis in transgenic C. elegans. Biotechniques 32(4):728–730

6. O'Halloran DM (2015) STITCHER: a web resource for high-throughput design of primers for overlapping PCR applications. Biotechniques 58(6):325

7. Lipman DJ, Pearson WR (1985) Rapid and sensitive protein similarity searches. Science 227(4693):1435–1441

8. Rychlik W, Rhoads RE (1989) A computer program for choosing optimal oligonucleotides for filter hybridization, sequencing and in vitro amplification of DNA. Nucleic Acids Res 17(21):8543–8551

9. Li K, Brownley A, Stockwell TB et al (2008) Novel computational methods for increasing PCR primer design effectiveness in directed sequencing. BMC Bioinformatics 9:191. doi:10.1186/1471-2105-9-191

10. Boulin T, Etchberger JF, Hobert O (2006) Reporter gene fusions. In: The *C. elegans* Research Community (ed) WormBook. WormBook. doi:10.1895/wormbook.1.106.1. http://www.wormbook.org

11. Allawi HT, SantaLucia J Jr (1997) Thermodynamics and NMR of internal G.T mismatches in DNA. Biochemistry 36(34):10581–10594. doi:10.1021/bi962590c

12. Untergasser A, Nijveen H, Rao X et al (2007) Primer3Plus, an enhanced web interface to Primer3. Nucleic Acids Res 35(Web Server issue):W71–W74, gkm306 [pii]

Chapter 2

Synthetic Gene Design Using Codon Optimization On-Line (COOL)

Kai Yu, Kok Siong Ang, and Dong-Yup Lee

Abstract

Codon optimization has been widely used for designing native or synthetic genes to enhance their expression in heterologous host organisms. We recently developed Codon Optimization On-Line (COOL) which is a web-based tool to provide multi-objective codon optimization functionality for synthetic gene design. COOL provides a simple and flexible interface for customizing codon optimization based on several design parameters such as individual codon usage, codon pairing, and codon adaptation index. User-defined sequences can also be compared against the COOL optimized ones to show the extent by which the user's sequences can be evaluated and further improved. The utility of COOL is demonstrated via a case study where the codon optimized sequence of an invertase enzyme is generated for the enhanced expression in *E. coli*.

Key words Synthetic gene design, Web application, Codon optimization, Synthetic biology

1 Introduction

Gene design has been a fast advancing area with the decreasing price for DNA synthesis. Optimizing existing or synthetic genes is potentially important to achieve a satisfactory level of gene expression, whose product is most often a functional protein. Every step related to gene expression, including transcription, translation, and post-translational modification, can have a considerable impact on the final yield of the protein product. Codon optimization through synonymous codon substitutions provides a strategy that aims to increase the speed of translation elongation, thus enhancing expression in a specific host. This strategy has been successfully demonstrated to significantly improve the expression of recombinant proteins [1].

Codon optimization arises from the codon usage bias which has been observed in many organisms, especially in lower level of life forms. Although the origin of these preferences is still debatable from the perspective of molecular evolution, it is generally acknowledged that organism-specific codon preferences reflect a

Randall A. Hughes (ed.), *Synthetic DNA: Methods and Protocols*, Methods in Molecular Biology, vol. 1472,
DOI 10.1007/978-1-4939-6343-0_2, © Springer Science+Business Media New York 2017

balance between mutational biases and natural selection for translational improvement or optimization [2]. To compute a host's codon usage for codon optimization, we can select all the genes in its genome, or a subset of genes (e.g., highly expressed genes) if these genes show a significantly different codon bias. The codon usage of an organism can be measured using indices such as the individual codon usage (ICU) or codon adaptation index (CAI). By replacing rare codons with the host's preferred codons, the translation speed can be potentially increased [3]. Codon pair or codon context (CC) has also been demonstrated to be relevant and implemented as an effective design criterion for codon optimization [4]. In addition to codon usage patterns, other factors such as mRNA stability and motifs such as hidden stop codons have been attributed to influence gene expression as well [5]. Therefore, multiple design factors should be considered simultaneously for better gene design. To do so, we developed Codon Optimization On-Line (COOL) as a web-based application for multi-objective codon optimization. COOL facilitates the design of a gene that is targeted to be expressed in a desired host organism by imitating the codon pattern of highly expressed genes in the hosts, and excluding undesired sequence motifs. Users can also visualize the scoring of the optimized sequences to compare trade-offs between different design criteria, as well as include user-defined sequences for comparison.

2   Materials

2.1 Gene Design Criteria

Three indices have been implemented in COOL to characterize the host codon usage pattern. The most popular index used is the CAI, which measures the deviation from the most frequently used synonymous codon of each amino acid. Another commonly used index is the ICU, which measures the frequency by which individual codons appear in a set of coding sequences. The CC index characterizes the nonrandom appearance of consecutive codon pairings. Other design criteria available are: GC content, exclusion sequences, repeat motifs, and hidden stop codons. These criteria can be used to fine-tune sequence design, such as removing restriction sites through the exclusion sequence criterion.

2.2 Algorithm

Effective gene design requires the consideration of multiple, possibly conflicting design factors. To address this, we recently implemented a multi-objective framework for codon optimization to handle such design problems [6]. The NSGAII multi-objective optimization program forms the heart of the framework [7]. Since we are optimizing gene sequences, the genetic algorithm based program is eminently suited for this task. Initially, the algorithm generates a population of nucleotide sequences with randomly selected synonymous codons that encode the same desired protein. The population size used scales with the input sequence length. For each specified optimization objective, the corresponding fitness value is computed for all sequences. Next, the sequences are compared among themselves and then sorted by Pareto domination, i.e., sequences that are superior to others in one or more objectives. Thereafter, the termination criterion is checked. The algorithm is set to terminate when the maximum number of iterations is reached. This limit scales with the population size. Following the termination check, the top half of the population is retained as parents to generate new solutions through genetic operators. Two parent sequences are randomly selected and combined via the crossover operation to generate two new child sequences. The child sequences then undergo random mutations to increase genetic diversity. This continues until the population has been refilled, and the fitness values of the selected objectives are computed for each new child sequence. The algorithm now continues to the next iteration where the population is checked for termination, ranked for elimination of inferior sequences, and the generation of new sequences. After the final iteration, the top half of final population is retained as solutions to be presented to the user.

2.3 Implementation

COOL is a web server built with the open-source LAMP solution stack (Linux, Apache, MySQL, PHP) based on a Model-View-Controller (MVC) architecture [8]. The multi-objective genetic algorithm [6] is implemented in C with interaction with a MySQL database via Perl scripts to read inputs and write results. COOL is freely available for academic and noncommercial users at http://bioinfo.bti.a-star.edu.sg/COOL/. The 32-bit Linux version of the program and sample input can be downloaded from the website under MIT license and WebMOCO license.

3 Methods

The web interface is built to be user-friendly and easy to follow. The codon optimization process can be fully customized through a step-by-step job submission process which allows users to specify their preferred parameter settings. After specifying the desired settings on the webpage for each step, the user can continue by clicking the "Save and Continue" button. Users can return to previous setup pages through the link tabs located near the top of the page to modify settings. Users have to click "Save and Continue" again for the modifications to be saved. The general workflow of COOL is illustrated in Fig. 1 and the details for each step are discussed in the following subsections.

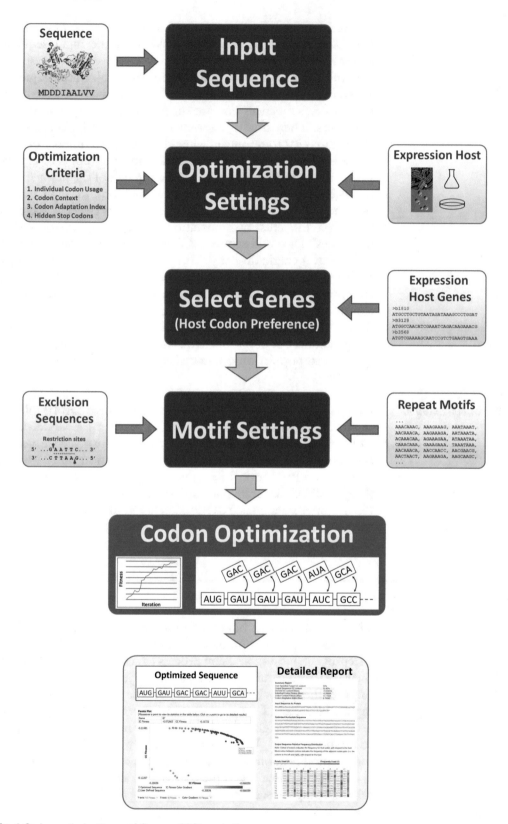

Fig. 1 Codon optimization workflow on COOL website

3.1 Input Sequence

From the homepage of the website, click on the "new job" link at the top of the page, or the "Start Using Codon Optimization On-Line link" to start. Either link will bring you to the "Input Sequence page". In this page, users have to enter the sequence to be codon optimized. First, select the sequence type, DNA/RNA or protein (*see* **Note 1**). For a nucleotide sequence, they will also have to select the relevant translation rules that apply to the input. The sequence must contain a start codon at the beginning and may contain one stop codon at the end of the sequence, conforming to the selected translation rules. The nucleotide sequence must not contain ambiguous bases (only ACGTU are permitted), and the total number of bases must be divisible by 3. For protein input, users must supply a sequence with a methionine start, and an optional termination signal (* or .) at the end. The human insulin and human beta actin sequences have been included on the webpage as samples for protein and DNA sequences respectively (Fig. 2). When either sample is selected, the respective sample sequence will be loaded into the input sequence textbox, and the process will automatically go to the next step.

1: Input Sequence	2: Optimization Settings	3: Select Genes	4: Motif Settings	5: Submit

Help

Select Input Type:

● **Protein**   Load Human Insulin Sample Protein Data

Note: A valid protein sequence should start with Methionine (M), and consists entirely of unambiguous amino acids (R, H, K, D, E, S, T, N, Q, C, G, P, A, V, I, L, M, F, Y, W). Please do not include the termination signal (*) or any other symbol.

○ **DNA/RNA**   Load Human Beta Actin Sample DNA Data

Note: A valid nucleotide sequence should start with Methionine (ATG/AUG), and end with a stop codon, with no other stop codons in the middle. It must consist entirely of unambiguous bases (A, C, G, T, U), and the number of bases should be divisible by 3. You must also select a translation code for your input sequence from the list below:

Standard Code	⏷

Enter Input Sequence:

This input sequence textbox accepts spaces and linebreaks that may be used to space out the sequence.

Optional: Enter a title for this sequence

Save And Continue

Fig. 2 Screenshot of the sequence input page

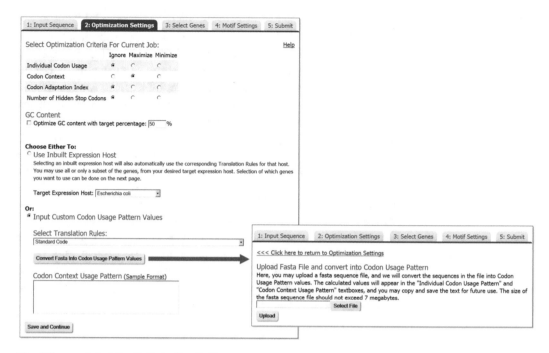

Fig. 3 Screenshot of the Optimization Settings page

Users have the option of giving a job title for the current job, which will be included in the output report. This is useful if users are submitting more than one sequence for optimization. When it is done, click "Save and Continue" to save the input and continue with the configuration process.

3.2 Optimization Settings

This page is the key step for selecting optimization parameters. The page is divided into three sections (Fig. 3). The four optimization criteria available in the first section are: Individual Codon Usage (ICU), Codon Context (CC), Codon Adaptation Index (CAI), and Number of Hidden Stop Codon (HSC). For each criterion, one can choose to maximize, minimize, or ignore it. At least one of these parameter should be active (maximize or minimize) to serve as a target for the optimization algorithm. *See* **Note 2** for a detailed explanation on these parameters.

In the second section, users can enable GC content as an optimization target. This field is useful if the optimized sequence should have a specific GC content value, such as the average GC content of the expression host, or of a particular gene. To enable GC content as an optimization criterion, ensure that the checkbox is ticked and enter the target as a percentage value (e.g., "38" instead of "0.38").

In the final section, users have to define the desired codon usage pattern(s) as the target for codon optimization. If the ICU or CAI criterion is active, the ICU pattern has to be specified, while

CC pattern has to be specified if the CC criterion is in use. There are two ways to specify the relevant codon usage patterns: using the inbuilt hosts, or user specified codon usage patterns. If users select an inbuilt expression host, the relevant translation rules will be automatically selected, and they will be asked to select the desired genes to generate the relevant codon usage pattern in the next step. The currently available hosts are *Escherichia coli*, *Lactococcus lactis*, *Pichia pastoris*, and *Saccharomyces cerevisiae*. Alternatively, users may specify your desired codon usage patterns manually, or upload their own set of genes in a .fasta formatted file (with a file size no larger than 7 MB) to compute the relevant codon usage patterns. To manually specify the codon usage pattern, each codon or codon pair should be entered into the relevant textboxes in capital letters, followed by the corresponding frequency counts separated by a space in each line (e.g., AAACAA 534 means the codon pair AAACAA has 534 occurrences). A sample file containing the format is available in a link beside the input textbox. If a set of genes is uploaded, the frequency counts of each codon and/or codon pairs will be computed and displayed in the Individual Codon Usage Pattern and/or Codon Context Usage Pattern dialogue boxes; these values can be modified by the user. Users will also have to specify here the appropriate codon translation rules that apply to sequence translation in the host (*see* **Note 3**). When it is done, click "Save and Continue".

3.3 Select Genes

If users have selected an inbuilt expression host in the previous page, they will be required to select genes from the host to compute the codon patterns (*see* **Note 4**). Otherwise, this page is unnecessary and will be skipped automatically. By default, all genes of the selected expression host are selected (Fig. 4). Users can enter their own list of gene locus tags into the "Input Quick Gene Selection List" textbox for genes that they wish to use instead. All recognizable genes that are on the list will appear in the "Selected Genes" list when users click "Select Genes from Text Input", while unrecognized entries will be placed in the "Unrecognized Gene ID List".

Users can also remove specific genes from the "Selected Genes" list by highlighting the gene and clicking "Remove Chosen Genes From Selected List". The removed genes will then be moved to the "Genes Available for Selection" list. Hold down the "Ctrl" key to select more than one gene. If users want to add any genes back, click on the genes and click the "Add Chosen Genes to Selected List" button. If any list on this page is hidden, click on the "Show List" link beside the list title to expand. The genes that appear in the "Selected Genes" list will be used to compute the codon usage patterns that are used as targets for the optimization criteria selected in the previous page. When the user is done with gene selection, click "Save and Continue". Alternatively, if users wish to change their expression host at this point in time, they can return

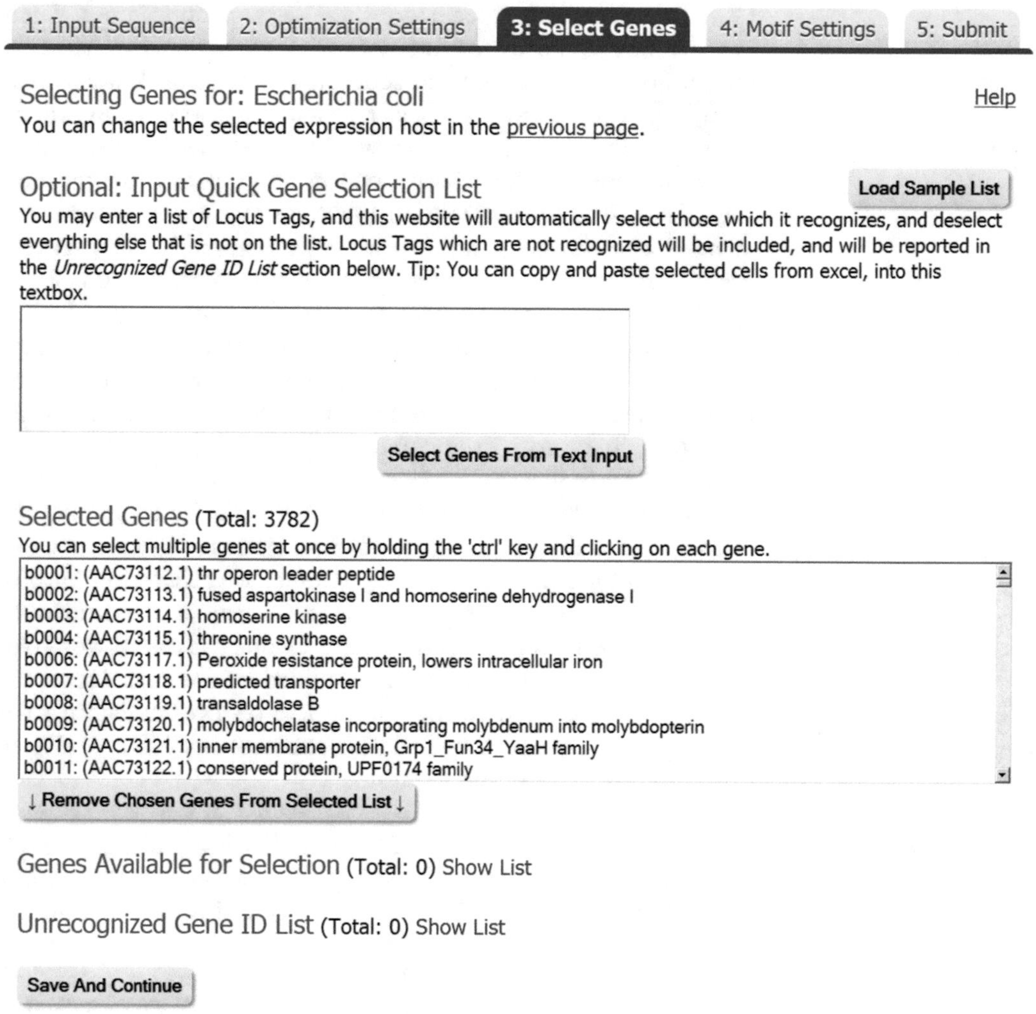

| 1: Input Sequence | 2: Optimization Settings | **3: Select Genes** | 4: Motif Settings | 5: Submit |

Selecting Genes for: Escherichia coli   Help

You can change the selected expression host in the previous page.

Optional: Input Quick Gene Selection List   Load Sample List

You may enter a list of Locus Tags, and this website will automatically select those which it recognizes, and deselect everything else that is not on the list. Locus Tags which are not recognized will be included, and will be reported in the *Unrecognized Gene ID List* section below. Tip: You can copy and paste selected cells from excel, into this textbox.

Select Genes From Text Input

Selected Genes (Total: 3782)

You can select multiple genes at once by holding the 'ctrl' key and clicking on each gene.

b0001: (AAC73112.1) thr operon leader peptide
b0002: (AAC73113.1) fused aspartokinase I and homoserine dehydrogenase I
b0003: (AAC73114.1) homoserine kinase
b0004: (AAC73115.1) threonine synthase
b0006: (AAC73117.1) Peroxide resistance protein, lowers intracellular iron
b0007: (AAC73118.1) predicted transporter
b0008: (AAC73119.1) transaldolase B
b0009: (AAC73120.1) molybdochelatase incorporating molybdenum into molybdopterin
b0010: (AAC73121.1) inner membrane protein, Grp1_Fun34_YaaH family
b0011: (AAC73122.1) conserved protein, UPF0174 family

↓ Remove Chosen Genes From Selected List ↓

Genes Available for Selection (Total: 0) Show List

Unrecognized Gene ID List (Total: 0) Show List

Save And Continue

Fig. 4 Screenshot of the gene selection page for *E. coli*

to the previous page via the link near the top of the page below the tabs and make the necessary change. After making the change(s), click "Save and Continue" to return to this page. The genes available for selection will reflect the change in expression host.

3.4 Motif Settings

There are two sections on this page (Fig. 5). In the "Exclusion Sequences" section, users can specify specific nucleotide sequences to be excluded from the final output. For example, users may want to remove the recognition sites of restriction enzymes that they intend to use for cloning. Users can select common restriction sites by name, from the drop-down menu bar (sorted alphabetically). By clicking on a restriction site name, its recognition sequence will be added into the textbox. One can also add their own sequences into the textbox. Each sequence should be at least four nucleotides long, contain unambiguous bases (ACGTU), and separated by a comma.

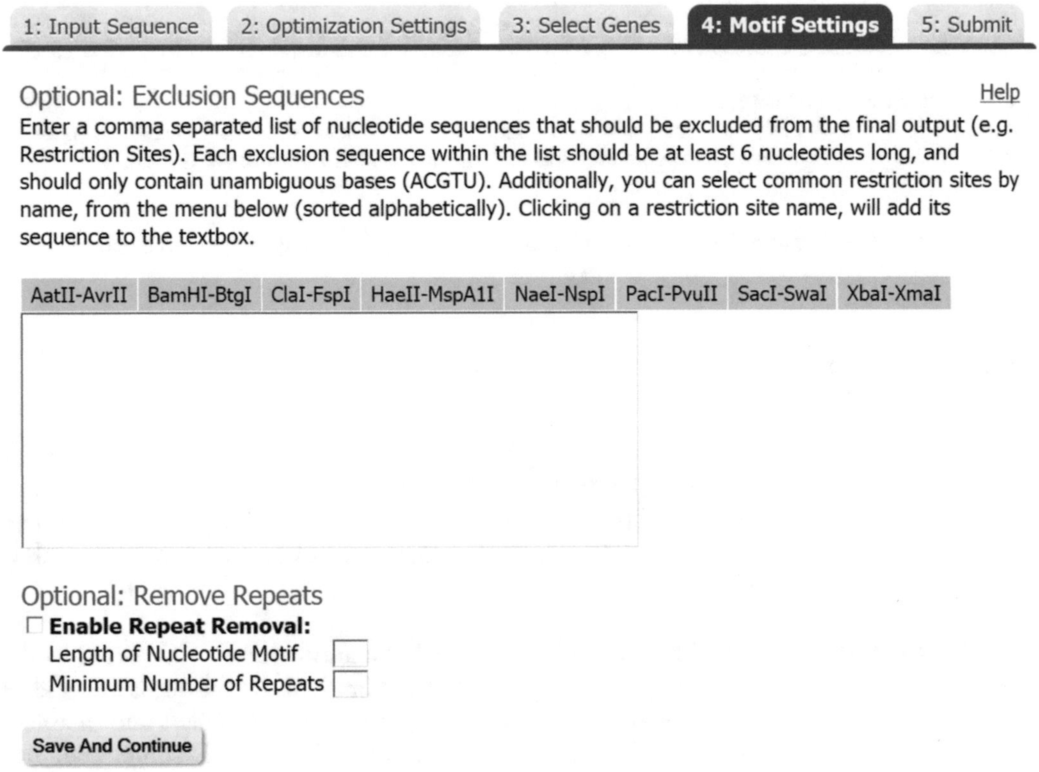

| 1: Input Sequence | 2: Optimization Settings | 3: Select Genes | **4: Motif Settings** | 5: Submit |

Optional: Exclusion Sequences   Help

Enter a comma separated list of nucleotide sequences that should be excluded from the final output (e.g. Restriction Sites). Each exclusion sequence within the list should be at least 6 nucleotides long, and should only contain unambiguous bases (ACGTU). Additionally, you can select common restriction sites by name, from the menu below (sorted alphabetically). Clicking on a restriction site name, will add its sequence to the textbox.

| AatII-AvrII | BamHI-BtgI | ClaI-FspI | HaeII-MspA1I | NaeI-NspI | PacI-PvuII | SacI-SwaI | XbaI-XmaI |

Optional: Remove Repeats
□ **Enable Repeat Removal:**
  Length of Nucleotide Motif ☐
  Minimum Number of Repeats ☐

[Save And Continue]

Fig. 5 Screenshot of the Motif Settings page

In the "Remove Repeats" section, users can enable repeats removal by specifying the "Length of Nucleotide Motif" and the "Minimum Number of Repeats". For example, if the "Length of Nucleotide Motif" is 2, this will include all possible $2^4 = 16$ dinucleotide motifs (AA, AT, AC, AG, TA, TT, TC, TG, CA, CT, CC, CG, GA, GT, GC, GG). If "Minimum Number of Repeats" is 3, then a particular motif must occur three or more consecutive times to be considered a repeat. Hence "ATATAT" would qualify. Both settings have a minimum of allowed value of 2. You must tick the "Enable Repeat Removal" box for this option to be active, or the length and number values will be ignored. Note that the algorithm is NOT guaranteed to remove all exclusion sequences and/or repeats, due to the encoded amino acid sequence (*see* **Note 5**).

3.5 Submit

This is the last page for setting up a job (Fig. 6). Users may enter their email address, and an automated notification email will be sent to the address when the results are ready to be viewed. An email address is not required but strongly encouraged for larger jobs, as the run may take more than a few minutes to complete. Users can use the link provided in the email to access the results for up to 1 month after job completion. Note that the automated notification email may trigger spam filters and be placed in the

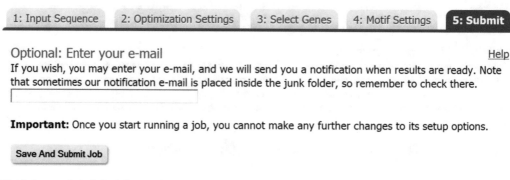

Fig. 6 Screenshot of the job submission page

spam folder. At this point, one may wish to review the selections by navigating to the previous pages through the links in the tabs near the top of the page. Click on "Save and Submit Job" button to launch the job. No further changes can be made once the job is submitted.

3.6 Check Results

After job submission, users will be automatically redirected to the results page. If the job is not yet finished, it will display a "Please Wait" message. If you have Java correctly installed and enabled, the page will refresh every minute until the job is completed. You can also bookmark the URL address of this page and check on your results at a later time. The waiting time depends on the length of the sequence. For a 500-amino acid sequence with all optimization criteria and motif settings active, the estimated time is about 8 min. Once the job is completed, the program displays the results, and sends the user a notification email with a link accessing the result page if an email address was provided earlier.

3.7 Results

When two or more optimization criteria have been selected, the optimized solutions will be depicted on a two-dimensional graph (Fig. 7) on the "Summary of Results" page. The optimized solutions should form a Pareto front, which depicts the trade-off between satisfying more than one optimization criteria (*see* **Notes 6** and **7**). The curve may not be smooth, especially if more than two optimization criteria were specified, since the solution space is compressed down to two dimensions. Users can also use the color coding of each point to serve as a third dimension for another optimization criterion. Users can switch the optimization criteria displayed on the axes and color coding via the drop-down menus below the Pareto plot. By mousing over a data point, the fitness values for each solution will be displayed on the mouse tooltips or statistics table above the graph; the exact behavior is browser dependent (*see* **Note 8**).

The optimized solutions are listed in a summary table below the Pareto plot. The fitness values of active optimization criteria for

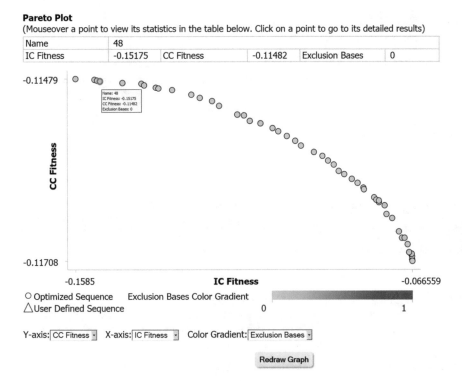

Pareto Plot

(Mouseover a point to view its statistics in the table below. Click on a point to go to its detailed results)

Name	48				
IC Fitness	-0.15175	CC Fitness	-0.11482	Exclusion Bases	0

Fig. 7 The Pareto plot

each solution are listed alongside, and you can click on the column headers to sort in ascending or descending order. Clicking on the name of a solution will lead you to its detailed report page, including the optimized sequence and its codon usage patterns. The detailed results can also be exported in the PDF format, and the optimized sequences may be exported to a tab-delimited file with fitness values. The exported PDF report contains the same information as the detailed report webpage, but without interactive features such as show/hide functions and sortable tables.

In the detailed report, there are several sections included (Fig. 8): the fitness scores of the active optimization criteria ("Summary Report"), the protein translation of the sequence ("Input Sequence As Protein"), the optimized nucleotide sequence ("Optimized Nucleotide Sequence"), codon usage of the sequence in relation to the host codon usage in color code ("Output Sequence Relative Frequency Distribution"), and detailed information for each active optimization criterion. The detailed information for each active optimization criterion is hidden by default. Click on the "Show Report" link beside each title to display them.

The "Output Sequence Relative Frequency Distribution" shows the nucleotide sequence separated into individual codons. If the ICU or CAI criterion is active, the codons are color coded with

Summary Report (Download this result as a PDF.)

Output Sequence GC content   57.36%

Individual Codon Fitness (Max) -0.081613

Codon Context Fitness (Max)   -0.1161   Open CC Comparison Graph in new window

Input Sequence As Protein (Click on textbox to select all):

MALWMRLLPLLALLALWGPDPAAAFVNQHLCGSHLVEALYLVCGERGFFYTPKTRREAEDLQVGQVELGGGPGAGSLQPLALEGSLQKRGIV
EQCCTSICSLYQLENYCN*

Optimized Nucleotide Sequence (Click on textbox to select all):

ATGGCGTTGTGGATGCGTCTGTTACCGCTGCTGGCATTGCTGGCGCTGTGGGGCCCGGACCCAGCCGCCGCGTTTGTCAACCAGCATCTGTG
CGGTTCTCACCTGGTGGAAGCCCTGTATCTGGTATGTGGCGAGCGTGGTTTCTTTTACACGCCGAAAACCCGCCGTGAAGCGGAAGATCTGC
AGGTGGGGCAGGTTGAACTGGGCGGCGGTCCTGGCGCAGGATCGCTGCAACCGCTCGCTCTTGAAGGTTCCTTACAAAAACGCGGCATTGTT
GAGCAGTGCTGCACCAGCATCTGTAGTCTTTATCAGCTGGAAAACTACTGCAATTAA

Output Sequence Relative Frequency Distribution

Note: Colour of codons indicates the frequency for that codon, with respect to the host. Block colour between codons indicates the frequency of the adjacent codon pairs (I.e. the codons to the left and right), with respect to the host.

Rarely Used (0)   **Frequently Used (1)**

Number:	1	2	3	4	5	6	7	8	9	10
1	ATG	GCG	TTG	TGG	ATG	CGT	CTG	TTA	CCG	CTG
11	CTG	GCA	TTG	CTG	GCG	CTG	TGG	GGC	CCG	GAC
21	CCA	GCC	GCC	GCG	TTT	GTC	AAC	CAG	CAT	CTG
31	TGC	GGT	TCT	CAC	CTG	GTG	GAA	GCC	CTG	TAT
41	CTG	GTA	TGT	GGC	GAG	CGT	GGT	TTC	TTT	TAC
51	ACG	CCG	AAA	ACC	CGC	CGT	GAA	GCG	GAA	GAT
61	CTG	CAG	GTG	GGG	CAG	GTT	GAA	CTG	GGC	GGC
71	GGT	CCT	GGC	GCA	GGA	TCG	CTG	CAA	CCG	CTC
81	GCT	CTT	GAA	GGT	TCC	TTA	CAA	AAA	CGC	GGC
91	ATT	GTT	GAG	CAG	TGC	TGC	ACC	AGC	ATC	TGT
101	AGT	CTT	TAT	CAG	CTG	GAA	AAC	TAC	TGC	AAT
111	TAA									

Fig. 8 Sample output page

its normalized appearance frequency in the host. If the CC criterion is active, the normalized codon pair appearance frequency of the host will be indicated by color-coded blocks appearing between successive codons. Below, the frequency and color tables for ICU and CC show the frequency of the codons/codon pairs in the host, as well as the optimized sequence in a table form. The "Host Vs Optimized Codon Relative Frequency Chart" also compares the codon/codon pair patterns of the host and the optimized sequence in a bar chart form.

If users have specified exclusion sequences and/or repeat motifs to be excluded from the optimized sequences, they have to view the "Exclusion Sequence Fitness" and/or "Repeat Fitness" sections of the report to check if these sequences are present in the sequence. The detailed reports for exclusion sequence fitness and repeat fitness will highlight the position of any unwanted sequence that appears in the optimized sequence, as well as list the appearance count of nucleotides from each exclusion sequence present.

Users can also compare the optimized nucleotide sequences generated by COOL with optimized sequences obtained from other sources. As a unique feature, user-defined DNA sequences (UDS) can be mapped onto the Pareto plot for comparison. They can add/delete UDS on the "Add/Remove User Defined Sequences" page (Fig. 9). This page can be accessed by clicking the "Add/Remove" link above the Pareto plot. Up to ten UDS can be added to each job for visualization. COOL will calculate the fitness values for the UDS, and add them to the summary table (and display them on the Pareto graph as well, if there are at least two optimization criteria). The relative positions of the user-defined sequences on the plot (shown with triangle symbols) will indicate their relative differences from the optimized sequences.

Add/Remove User Defined Sequences for: Human Insulin Sample Protein Data

<< Go Back to Results Summary   Help

Add New User Defined Nucleotide Sequence to Results:

A valid nucleotide sequence must consist entirely of unambiguous bases (A, C, G, T, U), and the number of bases should be divisible by 3. It should code for the protein sequence which was originally specified, using the translation rules of the expression host (Standard Code). This input sequence textbox also accepts spaces and linebreaks that may be used to space out the sequence.

Enter Title (Optional):

Add Sequence   **Add And Return to Summary**

Delete Existing User Defined Sequences

There are currently no User Defined Sequences

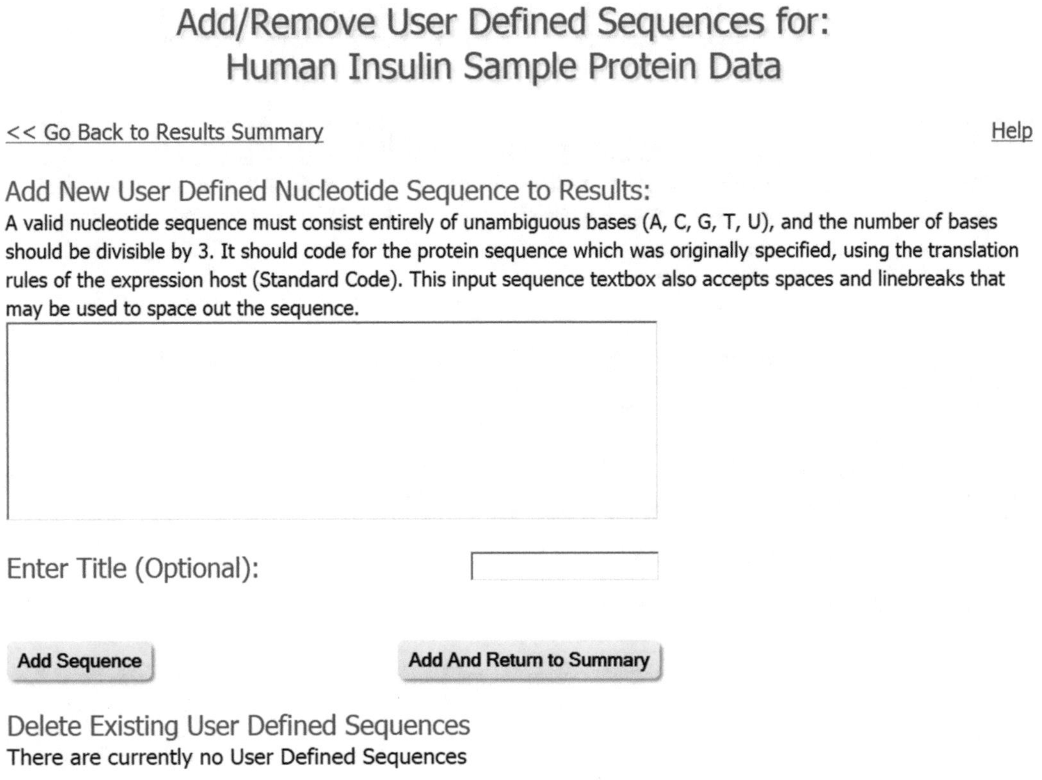

Fig. 9 Screenshot of the "Add/Remove User Defined Sequences" page

4   Case Study: Synthetic Gene Design of a Thermostable Invertase in *E. coli*

Here we give an example taken from a recently published codon optimization study [9]. The protein sequence to be optimized is beta-fructosidase (UniProt: O33833) or invertase from *Thermotoga maritima*, an enzyme that hydrolyzes sucrose to glucose and fructose. The protein sequence can be obtained from the UniProt website [10]. To express the protein, the common *E. coli* host is selected.

4.1   Input Sequence

Clicking on the "new job" link at the top of the page will start the process to configure a new codon optimization job with the "Input Sequence" page (Fig. 10). Since we have the protein sequence, we

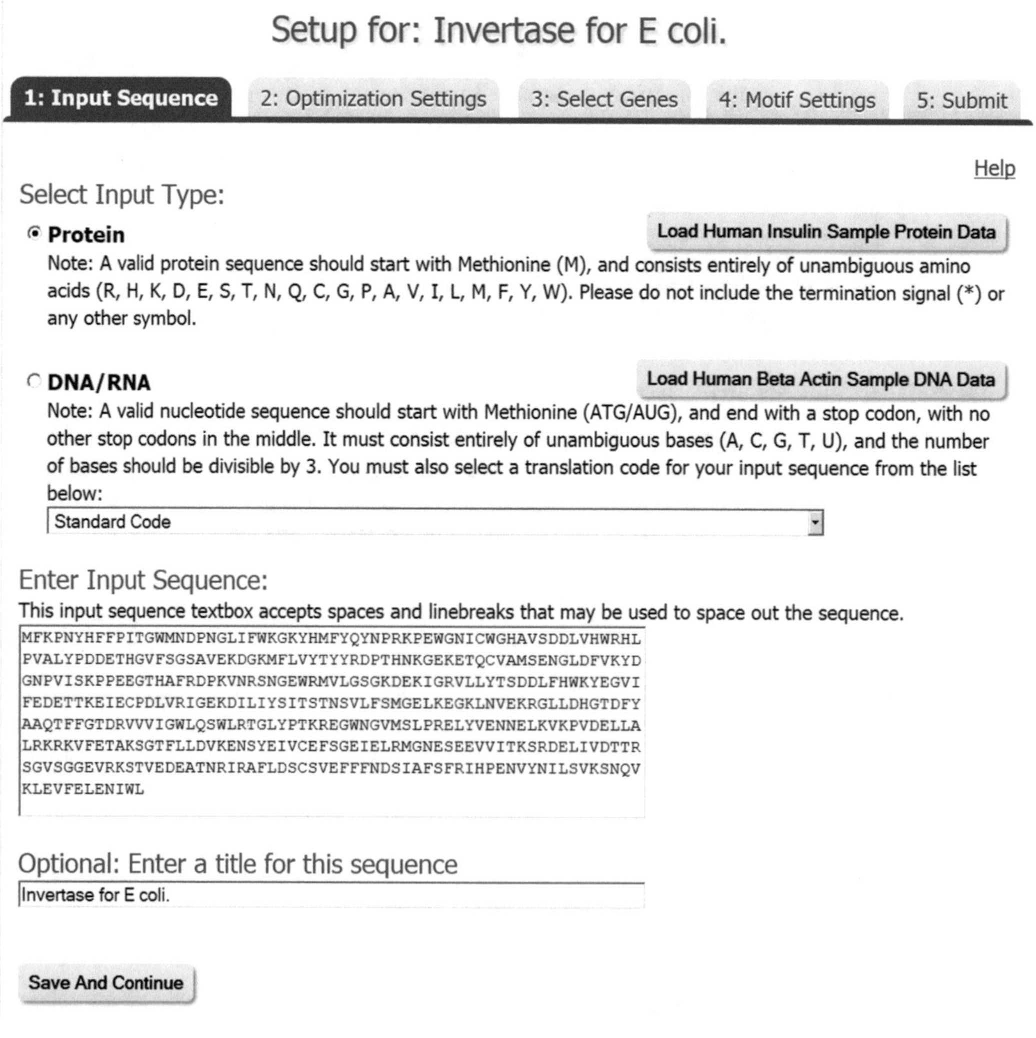

Setup for: Invertase for E coli.

| 1: Input Sequence | 2: Optimization Settings | 3: Select Genes | 4: Motif Settings | 5: Submit |

Help

Select Input Type:

◉ **Protein**   Load Human Insulin Sample Protein Data

Note: A valid protein sequence should start with Methionine (M), and consists entirely of unambiguous amino acids (R, H, K, D, E, S, T, N, Q, C, G, P, A, V, I, L, M, F, Y, W). Please do not include the termination signal (*) or any other symbol.

○ **DNA/RNA**   Load Human Beta Actin Sample DNA Data

Note: A valid nucleotide sequence should start with Methionine (ATG/AUG), and end with a stop codon, with no other stop codons in the middle. It must consist entirely of unambiguous bases (A, C, G, T, U), and the number of bases should be divisible by 3. You must also select a translation code for your input sequence from the list below:

| Standard Code   ▾ |

Enter Input Sequence:

This input sequence textbox accepts spaces and linebreaks that may be used to space out the sequence.

```
MFKPNYHFFPITGWMNDPNGLIFWKGKYHMFYQYNPRKPEWGNICWGHAVSDDLVHWRHL
PVALYPDDETHGVFSGSAVEKDGKMFLVYTYYRDPTHNKGEKETQCVAMSENGLDFVKYD
GNPVISKPPEEGTHAFRDPKVNRSNGEWRMVLGSGKDEKIGRVLLYTSDDLFHWKYEGVI
FEDETTKEIECPDLVRIGEKDILIYSITSTNSVLFSMGELKEGKLNVEKRGLLDHGTDFY
AAQTFFGTDRVVVIGWLQSWLRTGLYPTKREGWNGVMSLPRELYVENNELKVKPVDELLA
LRKRKVFETAKSGTFLLDVKENSYEIVCEFSGEIELRMGNESEEVVITKSRDELIVDTTR
SGVSGGEVRKSTVEDEATNRIRAFLDSCSVEFFFNDSIAFSFRIHPENVYNILSVKSNQV
KLEVFELENIWL
```

Optional: Enter a title for this sequence

| Invertase for E coli. |

Save And Continue

Fig. 10 Screenshot of the "Submit New Sequence" page for codon optimization of invertase

can copy and paste the sequence into the "Enter Input Sequence box". By entering a protein sequence, there is no need to select the codon translation rules for the sequence. We will give a title "Invertase for *E. coli*" to identify the job that we are submitting. We can now click on the "Save and Continue" button to go to the next page.

4.2 Optimization Settings

On the "Optimization Settings" page, we specify our desired optimization settings and host choice for this job (Fig. 11). In this case, we would like to consider two optimization criteria: ICU and CC. Therefore, we select to maximize both ICU and CC criteria. This way, the algorithm will generate the Pareto set of solutions that represent the trade-off between maximizing the ICU and CC criteria in the solutions. We do not activate the GC content option as we do not have a particular target for the GC content in this case. Since we are expressing the invertase enzyme in *E. coli*, we can use the "Use Inbuilt Expression Host" option with *E. coli*. We can now click the "Save and Continue" button to proceed with gene selection on the next page.

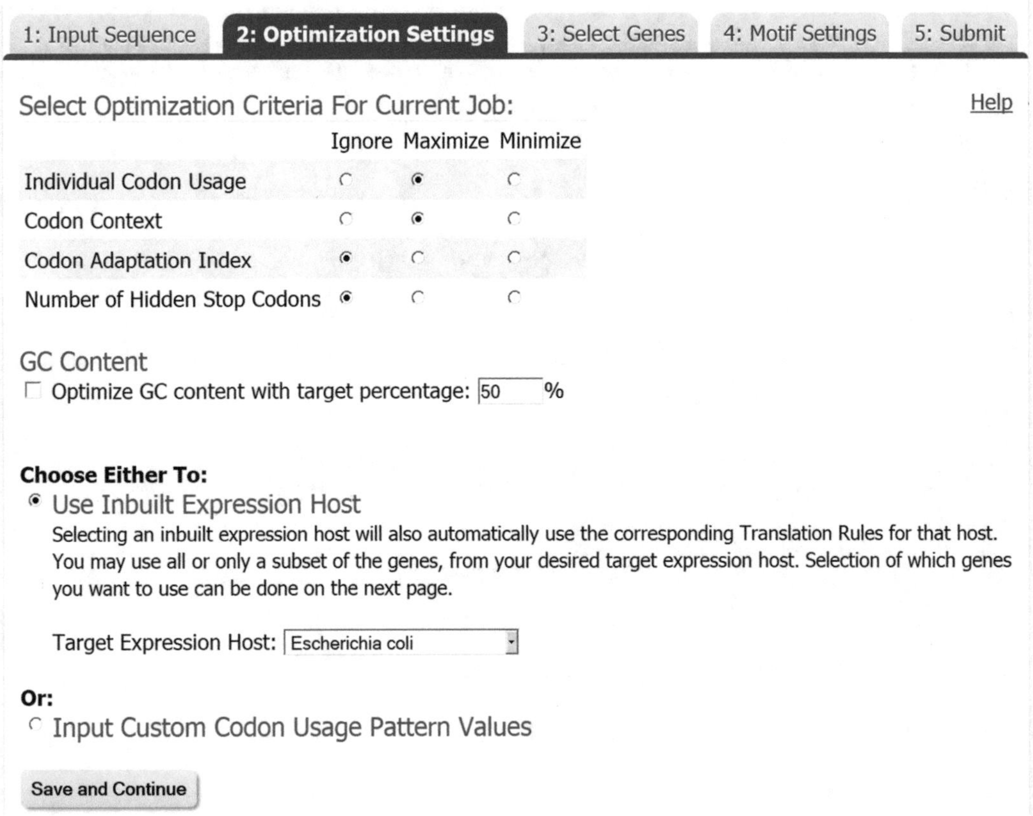

Fig. 11 Screenshot of the "Optimization Settings" page for codon optimization of invertase

4.3   *Select Genes*   Since we opted to use an inbuilt host, we have to select the genes of the host that are to be used to compute the codon bias (Fig. 12). By default, all genes are selected. However, in the published work [9], only the top 5 % highly expressed genes were used to compute the codon usage pattern; the locus tags of these genes are given in Table 1. We can copy and paste this set of locus tags into the "Input Quick Gene Selection List" input box and click the "Select Genes From Text Input" button. The website will recognize all 180 locus tags supplied and place them in the "Selected Genes" box. The remaining 3602 genes from the *E. coli* genome will now appear in the list of "Genes Available for Selection". We are now ready to proceed to the next page. Click the "Save and Continue" button.

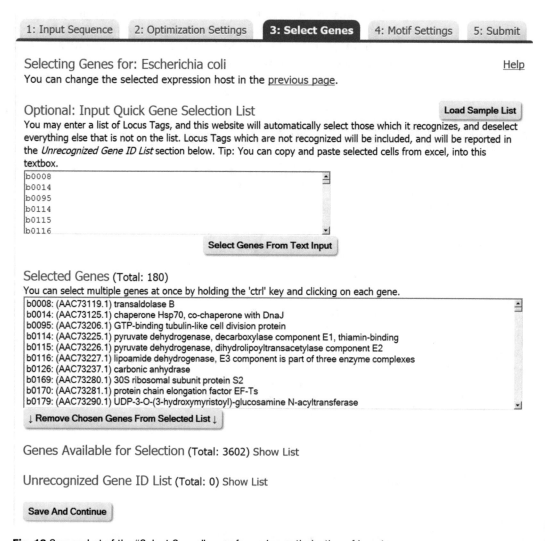

Fig. 12 Screenshot of the "Select Genes" page for codon optimization of invertase

Table 1
Locus tags of highly expressed genes of *E. coli* to be used for computing the codon usage pattern

b0008	b0741	b1092	b1779	b2417	b3097	b3304	b3342	b3781
b0014	b0742	b1093	b1818	b2478	b3098	b3305	b3357	b3829
b0095	b0755	b1094	b1823	b2528	b3169	b3306	b3433	b3936
b0114	b0811	b1101	b1824	b2572	b3186	b3307	b3460	b3983
b0115	b0812	b1136	b1920	b2597	b3212	b3308	b3495	b3984
b0116	b0814	b1237	b2007	b2606	b3213	b3309	b3510	b3985
b0126	b0880	b1243	b2029	b2607	b3230	b3310	b3610	b3986
b0169	b0884	b1324	b2093	b2608	b3231	b3311	b3636	b3987
b0170	b0889	b1480	b2094	b2609	b3236	b3312	b3637	b4000
b0179	b0903	b1583	b2095	b2696	b3255	b3313	b3649	b4014
b0197	b0911	b1603	b2096	b2697	b3261	b3314	b3672	b4015
b0220	b0912	b1641	b2175	b2741	b3294	b3315	b3703	b4142
b0407	b0928	b1656	b2185	b2742	b3295	b3316	b3730	b4171
b0474	b0929	b1677	b2215	b2779	b3296	b3317	b3733	b4172
b0525	b0953	b1712	b2285	b2780	b3297	b3318	b3734	b4200
b0565	b0957	b1713	b2296	b2891	b3299	b3319	b3735	b4201
b0605	b1051	b1716	b2323	b2904	b3300	b3320	b3737	b4202
b0623	b1088	b1717	b2414	b2913	b3301	b3321	b3738	b4243
b0727	b1089	b1719	b2415	b2926	b3302	b3340	b3751	b4245
b0728	b1091	b1761	b2416	b3065	b3303	b3341	b3766	b4255

4.4 Motif Settings

On the "Motif Settings" page (Fig. 13), we can specify the sequences or motifs that we wish to exclude from the optimized sequences. In this example, we wish to exclude the restriction sites of NcoI (CCATGG) and XhoI (CTCGAG). By mousing over the restriction site menus, they will expand and we can make our selections accordingly. In the event that the desired restriction sites are not available on the website, you can paste the sequence(s) into the textbox directly, separated by commas. In this example, there are no repeat motifs that we wish to exclude, so we will leave the "Remove repeats" option inactive. We can now click the "Save and Continue" button.

4.5 Submit

In this page before submitting the job, you can enter an email address to receive a notification upon job completion. You can also take the opportunity here to review the options selected in

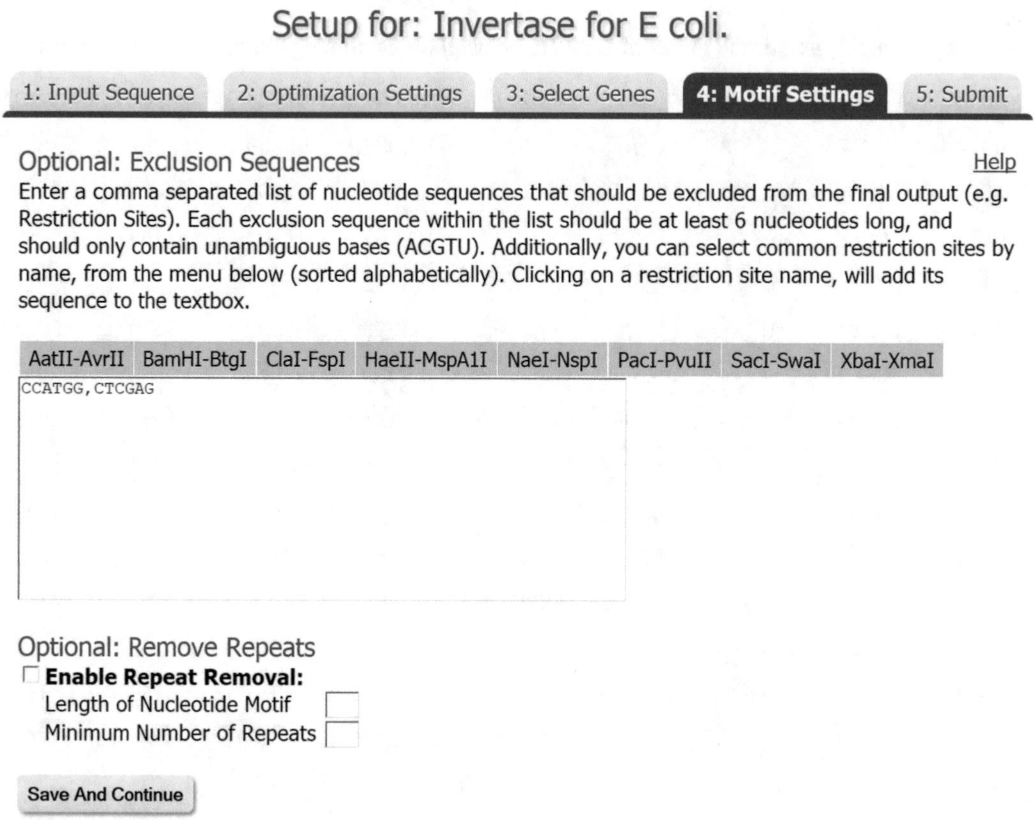

Setup for: Invertase for E coli.

| 1: Input Sequence | 2: Optimization Settings | 3: Select Genes | **4: Motif Settings** | 5: Submit |

Optional: Exclusion Sequences   Help

Enter a comma separated list of nucleotide sequences that should be excluded from the final output (e.g. Restriction Sites). Each exclusion sequence within the list should be at least 6 nucleotides long, and should only contain unambiguous bases (ACGTU). Additionally, you can select common restriction sites by name, from the menu below (sorted alphabetically). Clicking on a restriction site name, will add its sequence to the textbox.

| AatII-AvrII | BamHI-BtgI | ClaI-FspI | HaeII-MspA1I | NaeI-NspI | PacI-PvuII | SacI-SwaI | XbaI-XmaI |

```
CCATGG, CTCGAG
```

Optional: Remove Repeats
☐ **Enable Repeat Removal:**
Length of Nucleotide Motif ☐
Minimum Number of Repeats ☐

[Save And Continue]

Fig. 13 Screenshot of the "Motif Settings" page for codon optimization of invertase

the previous pages. Remember to click "Save and Continue" for any changes made. Once done, click "Save and Submit Job" to start the job.

4.6 Results

The optimization job for example should take approximately 3 min to complete. Upon completion, you can access the results through the link provided in the notification email (if you supplied an email address at the "Submit" page) or if you have kept the page open in the browser. By selecting two optimization criteria for this example, a Pareto plot will be shown. Since we have opted to exclude restriction sites from the optimized sequences, the number of exclusion bases appearing in the optimized sequences is depicted by the color coding on each plotted point. As the optimization algorithm is stochastic in nature, the results obtained will differ between different runs with the same protein product and optimization settings.

We can plot the position of the published codon context optimized sequence as an UDS using the "Add/Remove" link above the Pareto plot. When plotted, the added sequence will

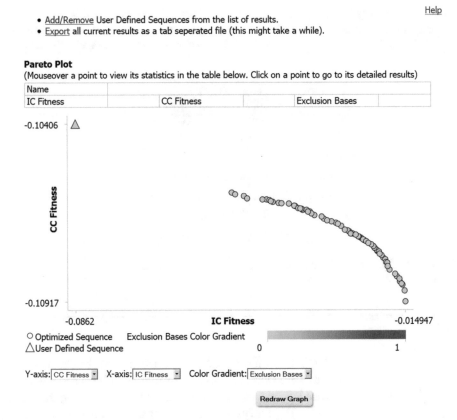

Summary of Results for: Your Target Sequence

Help

- Add/Remove User Defined Sequences from the list of results.
- Export all current results as a tab seperated file (this might take a while).

Pareto Plot
(Mouseover a point to view its statistics in the table below. Click on a point to go to its detailed results)

Name			
IC Fitness		CC Fitness	Exclusion Bases

○ Optimized Sequence   Exclusion Bases Color Gradient

△ User Defined Sequence

Y-axis: CC Fitness ▾   X-axis: IC Fitness ▾   Color Gradient: Exclusion Bases ▾

Redraw Graph

Fig. 14 Screenshot of the Pareto plot for codon optimization of invertase

appear as a triangle. The codon context optimized sequence will appear at top right corner of the Pareto plot, which denotes its high CC Fitness score but poor IC fitness score (Fig. 14). You can also add the wild-type sequence to the plot to see its difference from the optimized sequences in terms of IC and CC fitness. In addition to poor CC fitness, the wild-type sequence will also show poor CC fitness.

The detailed report for each optimized sequence is accessible via the table below the Pareto plot (Fig. 15). User added sequences will also appear in the table with the "UDS" prefix. Detailed reports for these sequences will be generated based on the optimization settings and are accessible just like the optimized sequences generated by the website. If we have only selected to optimize for the CC criterion, no Pareto plot will be shown and only this table will be displayed. The nucleotide sequence and detailed report for each solution can be accessed by the links on each table entry, with the pdf version alongside for saving to your PC.

Expression Host: Escherichia coli

If the Name starts with "UDS", that indicates that it is a User Defined Sequence. You can sort by a particular column, by clicking on the column header. Click once to sort ascending, and twice to sort descending. You can sort by multiple columns at once, by holding down 'shift' while clicking on the desired headers in order of sort priority.

Name (PDF)	IC Fitness (Max)	CC Fitness (Max)	Exclusion Bases
UDS: cco (pdf)	-0.0862	-0.10406	0
31 (pdf)	-0.052468	-0.10604	0
34 (pdf)	-0.051737	-0.10609	0
16 (pdf)	-0.049845	-0.10614	0
52 (pdf)	-0.049132	-0.10621	0
8 (pdf)	-0.044899	-0.10624	0

Fig. 15 Screenshot of the results table for codon optimization of invertase

5   Notes

1. No FASTA file-style header information should be included in the uploaded sequence. Numbers will be removed and lower-case letters will be automatically turned into capital letters. For DNA sequences, the length should be divisible by 3, and may end with an optional stop codon (no other in frame stop codons are allowed). If a problematic DNA sequence is uploaded, the program will reject the sequence and highlight the problem in an error message.

2. (a) ICU measures the appearance frequency of each codon, normalized by the frequency of the translated amino acid. When set to "Maximize", the optimization algorithm will modify the sequence to match the target ICU (e.g., the expression host's ICU). Conversely, the output sequence's ICU will be optimized to deviate from the host as much as it possible when set to "Minimize".

   (b) CC measures the appearance frequency of all possible codon pairs, normalized by the frequency of the translated amino acid pairs. Similar to ICU, a CC "Maximized" sequence will match the codon context pattern of the expression host as much as possible. The recommended default criterion is to Maximize Codon Context only.

   (c) CAI measures the synonymous codon that is most frequently encountered for each amino acid. When maximized, only the most frequent synonymous codon for each amino acid will be used.

(d) HSC refers to stop codons that are found in the +1 or –1 shifted reading frames. Selecting "Maximize" on "Number of Hidden Stop Codons", will maximize the number of hidden stop codons in the output sequence. This may be useful according to the ambush hypothesis, by causing erroneous frame-shifted translations to terminate early.

3. The translation rules you select here apply to the expression host, where the protein will be expressed. In contrast, the translation rules you selected back in **step 1**: Input Sequence, applies to the nucleotide sequence's original host, where the input nucleotide sequence was taken. For example, if you are trying to express a *Blepharisma* sequence in *Salmonella bongori* (which uses Standard translation rules), you should select "Standard Code" here.

4. The step for selecting the codon pattern of high-expression genes is only relevant if there are significant differences in the ICU and/or CC patterns between the average of all genes in the host's genome and a subset of genes (e.g., highly expressed genes). Otherwise, the ICU and CC patterns from the entire genome will be sufficient as the optimization target without the need to select highly expressed genes.

5. The program will try its best to remove all exclusion sequences and/or repeats, but there may be instances where this is simply not possible for the given protein sequence. Consider a protein with two consecutive methionine bases. This can only be coded in one way (ATGATG) under standard translation rules. If you specify "ATGATG" as an exclusion sequence, or that you want to remove repeats of three nucleotide motifs repeated two or more times (which includes ATGATG), the algorithm will be unable to meet your request. As such, the output results include count checks on whether any Exclusion Sequences or User-specified Repeats are present in the output sequence. Use these to check whether all Exclusion Sequences and Repeats are absent.

6. When more than one optimization criteria is specified, it is usually not possible to optimize for one criterion without sacrifices in other criteria. Therefore, a Pareto set of solutions can be computed to illustrate the trade-off in fitness between different criteria. When plotted, this Pareto set forms the Pareto front. For example, if you are trying to maximize both ICU and CC, the algorithm will produce a set of sequences. At one extreme, there will be a sequence with very high CC fitness, but very low ICU fitness. There will be other sequences with increasing ICU fitness, but decreasing CC fitness, until we reach the other extreme, with a sequence which has very high ICU fitness and very low CC fitness.

7. COOL optimizes the sequence based on the fitness values of the selected codon optimization criteria. However, these fitness values do not wholly predict the actual gene expression level that can be achieved. The exact roles played by individual optimization criteria as well as interaction effects have yet to be clearly elucidated. Furthermore, gene expression is regulated at multiple levels of transcription, translation, and post-translation. Thus there are a whole host of other factors, including noncoding regions that are outside the scope of codon optimization.

8. As the color coding is not a true axis dimension, we also allow users to plot values, which are not among the normal Pareto fitness parameters meant for the X/Y axis. Hence, beyond the four main optimization criteria on the "Optimization Settings" page, you may also choose to plot on the axes or color gradient: the GC content, the number of Exclusion bases, or the number of Repeat bases.

References

1. Elena C, Ravasi P, Castelli ME, Peiru S, Menzella HG (2014) Expression of codon optimized genes in microbial systems: current industrial applications and perspectives. Front Microbiol 5:21

2. Sharp PM, Li WH (1987) The codon adaptation index - a measure of directional synonymous codon usage bias, and its potential applications. Nucleic Acids Res 15:1281–1295

3. Makrides SC (1996) Strategies for achieving high-level expression of genes in Escherichia coli. Microbiol Rev 60:512–538

4. Chung BK-S, Yusufi FNK, Mariati YY, Lee D-Y (2013) Enhanced expression of codon optimized interferon gamma in CHO cells. J Biotechnol 167:326–333

5. Gould N, Hendy O, Papamichail D (2014) Computational tools and algorithms for designing customized synthetic genes. Front Bioeng Biotechnol 2:41

6. Chung BK-S, Lee D-Y (2012) Computational codon optimization of synthetic gene for protein expression. BMC Syst Biol 6:134

7. Deb K, Pratap A, Agarwal S, Meyarivan T (2002) Fast and elitist multiobjective genetic algorithm: NSGA-II. IEEE Trans Evol Comput 6:182–197

8. Chin JX, Chung BK-S, Lee D-Y (2014) Codon Optimization On-Line (COOL): a web-based multi-objective optimization platform for synthetic gene design. Bioinformatics 30: 2210–2212

9. Pek HB, Klement M, Ang K-S, Chung BK-S, Ow DS-W, Lee D-Y (2015) Exploring codon context bias for synthetic gene design of a thermostable invertase in Escherichia coli. Enzyme Microb Technol 75–76:57–63

10. The UniProt Consortium (2015) UniProt: a hub for protein information. Nucleic Acids Res 43(D1):D204–D212

Chapter 3

Shuffle Optimizer: A Program to Optimize DNA Shuffling for Protein Engineering

John N. Milligan and Daniel J. Garry

Abstract

DNA shuffling is a powerful tool to develop libraries of variants for protein engineering. Here, we present a protocol to use our freely available and easy-to-use computer program, Shuffle Optimizer. Shuffle Optimizer is written in the Python computer language and increases the nucleotide homology between two pieces of DNA desired to be shuffled together without changing the amino acid sequence. In addition we also include sections on optimal primer design for DNA shuffling and library construction, a small-volume ultrasonicator method to create sheared DNA, and finally a method to reassemble the sheared fragments and recover and clone the library. The Shuffle Optimizer program and these protocols will be useful to anyone desiring to perform any of the nucleotide homology-dependent shuffling methods.

Key words DNA shuffling, Codon optimization, Staggered extension process (StEP), Random chimeragenesis on transient templates (RACHITT), Protein library, Protein engineering, Computer program, Python

1 Introduction

In 1994, Dutch scientist Willem P.C. Stemmer invented a molecular breeding technique known as DNA shuffling [1]. Since that time, Stemmer's DNA shuffling method has been recognized as a powerful biotechnological tool and has been used to shuffle a panoply of DNA sequences coding for pharmaceutically relevant proteins, antibodies, biosynthetic pathways, viruses, and even bacterial genomes [2–7]. Since that time, other methods of DNA shuffling have emerged [8–10].

The goal of all of these DNA shuffling methods is to generate libraries of chimeric variants from the DNA of two or more related proteins, viruses, or bacteria which then can be subjected to functional screening or selection via directed evolution. The majority of these shuffling methods, including Stemmer's original method, rely on homology on the nucleic acid level to generate the chimeric constructs. Modeling and empirical data have additionally shown

Randall A. Hughes (ed.), *Synthetic DNA: Methods and Protocols*, Methods in Molecular Biology, vol. 1472,
DOI 10.1007/978-1-4939-6343-0_3, © Springer Science+Business Media New York 2017

that increased nucleic acid homology between the parental input constructs increases the frequency of crossing-over events in each chimera spawned, thus increasing library diversity [11, 12].

Here, we present Shuffle Optimizer, an easy-to-use python-based program to optimize regions of homology between two DNA sequences to be shuffled. This program will substitute synonymous codons in one sequence to increase the amount of DNA homology with the reference sequence without changing its amino acid sequence, thus increasing the number of crossovers and improving the shuffling procedure. While previous work has optimized sequences to shuffle based on free energy of annealing as well as homology, none of these programs are publically available or maintained, making implementation difficult [13, 14]. The Shuffle Optimizer program is written to run in the Python 2.7 programming language and requires the download and installation of the freely available Biopython suite of tools. The program runs quickly (less than one minute for a 1.8 kB gene), uses inputs of one nucleotide sequence to be optimized in relation to another, and outputs the optimized DNA sequence, a global protein alignment for those proteins, and metrics regarding the changes made to create the optimized sequence and the percent increase in homology resulting from optimization.

Here we present an example protocol to (1) obtain input sequences for Shuffle Optimizer, (2) install Python 2.7 and dependencies needed to run Shuffle Optimizer, (3) run Shuffle Optimizer, (4) design primers and constructs for DNA shuffling, and (5) perform DNA shuffling with the optimized construct. This example utilizes the original Stemmer method of DNA shuffling while using a DNA shearing ultrasonicator to create fragments of a specific size with high precision. This program should also aid those using less precise DNA fragmentation methods such as restriction enzyme or DNAse I-based fragmentation for the Stemmer DNA shuffling method. Similarly, Shuffle Optimizer could be used to aid other nucleic acid homology-based DNA shuffling methods beyond the original Stemmer method, such as the staggered extension process (StEP) and random chimeragenesis on transient templates (RACHITT) methods [8, 9].

In summary, Shuffle Optimizer optimizes homology by taking one input DNA sequence to be optimized and changing the codon sequence (but not the amino acid sequence) in order to increase the runs of perfect homology with the other input sequence, termed the reference sequence (*see* **Note 1**). This is done by taking the two input nucleic acid sequences, translating them, and performing a global alignment on the protein sequences (*see* **Note 2**) After global alignment, gaps are added to each nucleotide sequence matching the gaps in the global protein alignment. At this point, the program goes through each codon, starting with the first, and determines if the codons are matches or mismatches (gaps in either strand are ignored). Matches get passed over, leaving mismatches to be in one of two categories: (1) mismatches of the same amino acid (e.g.,

Lys-AAA and Lys-AAG) or (2) mismatches of different amino acids (e.g., Lys-AAA vs AAT-Asn). When the amino acids are the same, the program will change the optimized sequence to match the reference codon (e.g., from above, would add AAA instead of AAG if AAA was in the reference sequence). It has previously been assumed that annealing rarely occurs if sequence homology is <5 base pairs and occurs well when the sequence homology is >10 base pairs [11, 14]. As such, the program attempts to change the mismatched codon to another codon which still codes for that amino acid and increases the homology to either (or both) sides (*see* **Note 3**). When the program gets to the end of the global alignment it outputs the optimized sequence and a number of other metrics about how the optimization took place (*see* **Note 4**).

2   Materials

2.1   *For Running Shuffle Optimizer*

1. Download Python. The most 'recent Python 2.7 versions depend on whether a Mac/Linux or Windows OS machine is used (https://www.python.org/downloads/).

2. Download Biopython and NumPy (http://biopython.org/wiki/Download).

3. Download Shuffle Optimizer python program (https://sites.google.com/site/dnashufflingopt/home/code).

2.2   *For Shearing*

1. Covaris S2 ultrasonicator.

2. microTUBE AFA Fiber Snap-Cap tubes.

2.3   *For DNA Shuffling and General Reagents*

1. Platinum Taq HiFi DNA polymerase (Invitrogen).

2. PCR reagents (polymerase, dNTPs, buffer, 50 mM $MgSO_4$) (usually supplied with DNA polymerase).

3. Gel Purification/PCR Cleanup Kit.

4. Miniprep kit.

5. High-efficiency electrocompetent cells for cloning (i.e., Top10 from Invitrogen, DH10B, etc.).

6. Media for culturing *E. coli* (LB, 2XYT, or other standard media).

7. Agarose for making plates.

8. Petri Dishes.

9. Electrophoresis grade agarose.

10. Standard agarose gel electrophoresis equipment.

11. Plasmid backbone for cloning shuffled genes.

12. Selective antibiotic stocks (varies based on desired organism for library expression).

13. Nanodrop spectrophotometer.

3   Methods

3.1   Starting Sequence Considerations

To begin, one must decide what sequences to shuffle. Typically, the researcher already has an idea of what sequences they would like to shuffle based on homology modeling or independent research. One can also use Blastp (NCBI, http://blast.ncbi.nlm.nih.gov/Blast.cgi?PROGRAM=blastp&PAGE_TYPE=BlastSearch&LINK_LOC=blasthome) to identify potential candidates for shuffling by inputting a reference protein sequence. Shuffling of sequences with 43–48 % identities on the nucleotide level and 60–65 % homology on the protein level prior to optimization have been experimentally validated using the Shuffle Optimizer program, though this is not necessarily a lower limit.

In theory, one can use either protein sequences or DNA sequences of the desired genes as inputs for shuffling; codon optimization for optimal organism expression, outlined in methods, can be performed from either type of input. In practice, one typically has a DNA construct already built containing one of the sequences, which is ideally already codon optimized for the organism of choice. In this case, one can optimize all other sequences to this sequence to minimize the number of constructs one must build.

3.2   Obtaining Sequences for Shuffle Optimizer Input

1. Begin with sequences of the two genes of interest. DNA sequences should begin with a start codon (ATG) and end with a stop codon (TAA, TAG, or TGA). Only the coding sequence should be included; exclude introns. Protein sequences should begin with a methionine.

2. Perform codon optimization for efficient expression in the organism of choice on the desired input sequences (*see* **Note 5**). To do this, open a web browser and navigate to http://www.idtdna.com/CodonOpt (*see* **Note 6**). Select DNA Bases or Amino Acids as appropriate. Paste one sequence in the provided text box, and select the organism in which the experiment will be performed (e.g., *Escherichia coli*). Click Submit.

3. Copy one DNA sequence into a text file or preferred sequence software (*see* **Note 7**). Label the sequence and save the file for reference. If a protein sequence was used as an input, add a stop codon to the 3′ end of the DNA sequence.

4. Repeat **step 3** as necessary to codon optimize all desired sequences for the desired experimental organism. One should now have DNA sequences for all of the variants to be shuffled, beginning with a start codon and ending with a stop codon.

3.3   Running Shuffle Optimizer

1. **Windows Users**: Once Python and the appropriate modules have been obtained (*see* Subheading 2.1), open the python GUI (IDLE or equivalent, *see* Subheading 2.1), open the Shuffle Optimizer Module (File > Open, select Shuffle Optimizer), and

run the Module (Run > Run Module). The screen should display "Please input the reference DNA sequence."

Mac/Linux Users: Once Python and the appropriate modules have been obtained (*see* Subheading 2.1), open a terminal window, navigate to the file with "shuffleoptimizer.py" and type in "python shuffleoptimizer.py" to run the program. The screen should display "Please input the reference DNA sequence."

2. Copy the reference DNA sequence from the text file or sequence software and paste it into the program. **Important**: The DNA sequence must be pasted into the program as a single line with no line breaks, or the program will only read the first line. If pasting from sequence software, this is usually automatic; if pasting from notepad or other text files, the line breaks must be deleted (*see* **Note 8**). Hit enter. The display should now say "Please input the DNA sequence to be optimized."

3. Copy the DNA sequence to be optimized and paste it into the program. **Important**: The DNA sequence must be pasted into the program as a single line with no line breaks, or the program will only read the first line. If pasting from sequence software, this is usually automatic; if pasting from notepad or other text files, the line breaks must be deleted. Hit enter. The program will output the optimized DNA sequence, as well as several statistics about the optimization.

4. Copy the optimized DNA sequence and paste it into a text file or preferred sequence software. Label and save the sequence.

5. If desired, repeat **steps 1** through **4** for the other sequences to be shuffled. Use the same sequence as a reference in **step 2** for all optimizations performed.

3.4 Designing Primers and Constructs for DNA Shuffling

1. Obtain dsDNA corresponding to each of the gene sequences desired for shuffling. These can be synthesized as a single piece of DNA when ordered from most DNA synthesis companies, cloned from plasmids or genomes already containing the gene in the case of the reference sequence, or assembled via overlap PCR or similar methods.

2. Design and clone each gene to be shuffled into the preferred plasmid backbone for expression of the shuffled library in downstream screening or selection experiments using Gibson cloning, restriction cloning, or any other preferred method. There must be one construct per gene, and all constructs must contain the gene in the same exact location on the plasmid backbone.

3. Design a set of PCR primers to use for amplifying the genes to be shuffled from the constructs in **step 2**. Each primer should bind 200–300 base pairs outside the coding sequence on the vector backbone, such that an approximately equal=number of nucleotides is added to each side of the gene in the resulting

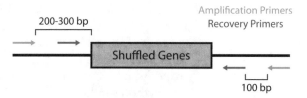

Fig. 1 Primer design for DNA Shuffling. The amplification primers, used to amplify DNA from all genes for shuffling, are pictured in *blue*, and should be 200–300 base pairs away from the gene. The recovery primers, used to recover the shuffled library from the reassembly reaction, are pictured in *red*, and should be at least 100 base pairs closer than the amplification primers to the gene

PCR (*see* Fig. 1, Blue). The same primers (herein, called amplification primers) can be used to amplify each gene to be shuffled, so only one set is needed.

4. Design a set of PCR primers (herein, called recovery primers) to recover shuffled gene products after the shuffling reaction. These primers should bind to the backbone between the amplification primers from **step 3** and the genes of interest, and be at least 100 base pairs closer to the gene of interest than the amplification primers (*see* **Note 9**) (*see* Fig. 1, Red).

5. Design primers for sequencing the individually cloned genes to be shuffled (from **step 2**) as well as for sequencing the shuffled library to be created if desired. This can be accomplished using a single set of primers ~50 bp outside the gene facing toward the gene, provided the gene is small enough and that typical Sanger sequencing yields are of sufficient length (*see* **Note 10**).

6. Sequence all constructs created in **step 2** using Sanger sequencing with primers from **step 5** before continuing to the DNA shuffling procedure to verify that sequences are correct for shuffling.

3.5 DNA Shuffling

1. Amplify each gene to be shuffled in separate PCRs using the amplification primers from Subheading 3.4, **step 3** (*see* **Note 11**).

2. Gel purify each gene desired for shuffling to remove primers and nonspecific products using any gel purification kit.

3. Add 5 μg total of DNA to a fresh tube. Typically, one would add equal amounts of DNA for each gene to be shuffled, but these ratios can be modified to bias certain genes in the subsequent reassembly reaction. For example, if there are two genes to be shuffled, add 2.5 μg of each for an unbiased shuffling.

4. Bring the total volume of the mixture up to 130 μL with water.

5. Transfer the mixture to a microAFA tube by sticking the pipette tip all the way to the bottom of the tube through the top opening; when pipetting the mixture in, slowly remove the tip to ensure loading the tube completely without air bubbles.

6. Load the tube into the tube holder and place in the water bath. Shear the DNA using the Covaris S2 ultrasonicator. Refer to the appropriate protocol at http://covarisinc.com/resources/protocols/ for details. For best results, shear DNA to between 100 and 200 base pairs in length. A typical program for 150 base pair fragments consists of the following settings:

   – Duty Cycle: 10%

   – Intensity: 5

   – Cycles per burst: 200

   – Time: 430 s

   (see Note 12)

7. Remove the tube. With the pipette depressed, stick the pipette tip into the top opening such that it is just below the top of the liquid. Slowly withdraw the DNA mixture, moving the pipette tip down toward the bottom of the tube, until all of the mixture is removed. Pipette into a fresh microtube.

8. Nanodrop the mixture to confirm concentration of the DNA. Be sure to label and save this tube for later analysis.

9. Set up the reassembly PCR. This PCR contains no primers. The mixture should contain:

   10 µL 10× Platinum Taq Hifi buffer

   5 µL 4 mM dNTP mixture (or equivalent)

   4 µL 50 mM MgSO4

	Temperature [C]	Time [m:s]
1.	95	2:00
2.	95	0:30
3.	65	1:30
4.	62	1:30
5.	59	1:30
6.	53	1:30
7.	50	1:30
8.	47	1:30
9.	44	1:30
10.	41	1:30
11.	68	1 min/kb
Go to step 2 (95 for 0:30) and repeat 2–11 for 35 total cycles		

0.4 µL Platinum Taq Hifi

200–500 ng sheared DNA from the sonicator

Up to 100 µL with ddH$_2$O

(see Note 13)

10. Run the PCR reaction with the preceding protocol on a thermal cycler. The extension time should be 1 min per kilobase of gene length of the longest gene included in the shuffling procedure.

11. Column purify the PCR reassembly reaction (**steps 9–10**) using a PCR cleanup kit.

12. Nanodrop the mixture to confirm concentration of the DNA. Be sure to label and save this tube for later analysis.

13. Set up a PCR reaction in quadruplicate using standard PCR conditions as specified by the supplier of the DNA polymerase used with 0–50 ng of purified DNA from **step 12**, the recovery primers from Subheading 3.4, **step 5**, and 20 cycles of amplification (*see* **Note 14**).

14. Run an agarose gel of the PCRs from **step 13** (entire reactions), the reassembly reaction from **step 12** (15–25 µL), and the sheared DNA from **step 8** (25–35 µL), using a relevant ladder with sizes spanning from the length of the sheared DNA (100–200 base pairs) to the length of the shuffled genes. The sheared DNA should appear as a smear centered around the size of the fragments the protocol used was targeting. The reassembly reaction should appear as a band or smear with the brightest section appearing around the average size of the shuffled genes. The recovery PCRs should contain a bright band around the average size of the shuffled genes.

15. Gel purify the reassembly PCRs using any DNA gel purification kit. Measure the concentration of shuffled DNA using a Nanodrop.

16. Clone the DNA into the preferred plasmid backbone for library expression and screening/selection in the desired organism. Typically, this is done using restriction/ligation cloning to achieve the highest possible yields, though other methods such as Gibson assembly may be used. Typically, 1 µg of backbone is used, with a 2:1 ratio of insert:backbone (*see* **Note 15**).

17. Column purify the cloning reaction using either a miniprep kit or a PCR cleanup kit.

18. Using all of the DNA from **step 17**, transform the cloned library into 100 µL of electrocompetent cells prepared from a high efficiency cloning strain of *E. coli* such as Top10 (Invitrogen) following the recommended electroporation conditions of the cell supplier (*see* **Note 16**).

19. After the 1 h recovery step in 1 mL of media in the transformation procedure, serial dilute a 100 µL aliquot of the cells 1:10 in 1 mL of fresh media 5–6 times (i.e., 100 µL of cells in

900 μL of media per dilution). Plate 100 μL of each dilution on plates containing the antibiotic corresponding to the resistance marker on the plasmid backbone.

20. Start a liquid culture of the library by diluting the remaining transformed library cells 1:10 into liquid media plus the antibiotic corresponding to the resistance marker on the plasmid backbone.

21. Grow all the plates and the liquid culture overnight.

22. Count colonies on the appropriate dilution plate; the plate should contain approximately 200 colonies. Multiply the number of colonies times the dilution factor (i.e., 10^5 for the fifth serial dilution) times 10 (plating 100 μL of cells is essentially another serial dilution). This is the theoretical yield of the library.

23. If desired, 10–20 colonies can be individually cultured in media plus selective antibiotic overnight and individually miniprepped and sequenced in order to investigate the efficiency of the shuffling procedure. Sequencing primers should bind to the plasmid backbone ~50 base pairs outside of the gene, facing inward (*see* Subheading 3.4, **step 5**).

24. Using a standard mini or midiprep kit, purify the plasmid DNA from the entire overnight liquid culture; this can be split across several minipreps. The library is now ready for transformation into the desired organism.

4   Notes

1. The program is not set up to optimize two sequences at the same time. As such, if one wanted to synthesize two optimized sequences in relation to one another, it is possible to run the program to optimize one sequence (e.g., unoptimized sequence A) in relation to the other (sequence B) then taking that optimized sequence (optimized sequence A) and running it as a reference while optimizing the other sequence (running unoptimized sequence B with optimized sequence A as the reference). This strategy offers a slight increase in homology between the sequences, but is generally not necessary.

2. The global alignment is performed by the Pairwise2 function in Biopython. It is currently set up to use the Clustal62 matrix, with a gap open penalty of -12 and a gap extend penalty of -3 (end gaps are not penalized). Depending on the length and homology between the two sequences, it may be desirable to change the Clustal matrix or the values of these gap open/extend penalties. This will require basal programming knowledge; however these parameters are clearly indicated in the code.

3. Specifically, if there is homology between 5 and 10 on both sides, the program attempts to add homology to whichever side is closer to 6 first. Then, if homology on a side is <6, the

program adds to the larger side. Otherwise, if the length of homologies are both >10, the program tries to add homology to the left side then to the right side.

4. The program outputs the aligned protein sequences translated from the input strings, the number of mismatches, the optimized sequence, the number of matched amino acids in the protein alignment changed to match the reference DNA codons, the number of matched amino acid codons changed in total, the number of mismatched amino acids not changed (and those which were already optimal), the number of codons optimized to add homology to the 3′ end, the number of codons optimized to add homology to the 5′ end, the number of total nucleotides changed and the percentage by which the homology was improved, and the percentage of total nucleotide homology between the reference sequence and the new optimized sequence.

5. If one of the gene sequences is already contained on a plasmid, PCR fragment, or genome, one need not optimize it; this may be used as the reference sequence in the shuffling program, to which other sequences will be optimized.

6. This is not the only available software for codon optimization; other resources may be used, if desired.

7. Multiple sequence outputs can be copied from the IDT codon optimizer, if desired, but the results are typically similar between variants.

8. The "reference" DNA sequence is not changed when running Shuffle Optimizer; if a construct is already built with one of the DNA sequences at this point, use this as the reference sequence.

9. Keep the downstream library cloning strategy in mind when designing these primers; if the intent is to use restriction cloning to create the shuffled library, make sure this PCR product will contain the desired restriction sites with enough overhang for proper cutting. If the intent is to use Gibson cloning, design an additional set of primers to amplify the backbone such that an overlap of ~30 base pairs exists between the recovered gene product and the amplified backbone.

10. While sequencing primers for individual genes may bind within the gene sequence, it is impossible to know which internal primers to use for shuffled variants without first sequencing with primers that bind to the backbone; for this reason, it is ideal to attempt to cover the full sequence length with primers that bind the backbone.

11. 5 μg total of DNA is needed for shuffling; for two gene shuffling, 2.5 μg of each gene fragment is needed, for example. Keep this in mind when setting up these PCRs, as multiple PCRs may be needed for each fragment to obtain this high yield.

12. It is critical that the water level, degassing level, and temperature are maintained at appropriate levels to prevent damaging the equipment and obtain adequate shearing results. Read the full protocol before proceeding.

13. It is critical that this reaction is run with Platinum Taq Hifi, available from Invitrogen, to ensure proper reassembly of the fragmented DNA.

14. This PCR does not require the use of Platinum Taq Hifi.

15. If ligating the insert into the backbone, be sure to treat the cut backbone with Calf Intestinal Phosphatase (CIP, New England Biolabs) to prevent self-ligation. If using Gibson assembly, the backbone can be amplified using PCR; be sure to treat the resulting reaction with DpnI (New England Biolabs) to ensure removal of plasmid before assembling.

16. For highest efficiency, transform the reaction using electro-competent cells. Freshly made electrocompetent cells will result in even higher transformation efficiency.

References

1. Stemmer WP (1994) DNA shuffling by random fragmentation and reassembly: in vitro recombination for molecular evolution. Proc Natl Acad Sci U S A 91(22):10747–10751

2. Chang CC, Chen TT, Cox BW, Dawes GN, Stemmer WP, Punnonen J, Patten PA (1999) Evolution of a cytokine using DNA family shuffling. Nat Biotechnol 17(8):793–797. doi:10.1038/11737

3. Crameri A, Raillard SA, Bermudez E, Stemmer WP (1998) DNA shuffling of a family of genes from diverse species accelerates directed evolution. Nature 391(6664):288–291. doi:10.1038/34663

4. Patten PA, Howard RJ, Stemmer WP (1997) Applications of DNA shuffling to pharmaceuticals and vaccines. Curr Opin Biotechnol 8(6):724–733

5. Powell SK, Kaloss MA, Pinkstaff A, McKee R, Burimski I, Pensiero M, Otto E, Stemmer WP, Soong NW (2000) Breeding of retroviruses by DNA shuffling for improved stability and processing yields. Nat Biotechnol 18(12):1279–1282. doi:10.1038/82391

6. Soong NW, Nomura L, Pekrun K, Reed M, Sheppard L, Dawes G, Stemmer WP (2000) Molecular breeding of viruses. Nat Genet 25(4):436–439. doi:10.1038/78132

7. Zhang YX, Perry K, Vinci VA, Powell K, Stemmer WP, del Cardayre SB (2002) Genome shuffling leads to rapid phenotypic improvement in bacteria. Nature 415(6872):644–646. doi:10.1038/415644a

8. Zhao H, Giver L, Shao Z, Affholter JA, Arnold FH (1998) Molecular evolution by staggered extension process (StEP) in vitro recombination. Nat Biotechnol 16(3):258–261. doi:10.1038/nbt0398-258

9. Coco WM, Levinson WE, Crist MJ, Hektor HJ, Darzins A, Pienkos PT, Squires CH, Monticello DJ (2001) DNA shuffling method for generating highly recombined genes and evolved enzymes. Nat Biotechnol 19(4):354–359. doi:10.1038/86744

10. O'Maille PE, Bakhtina M, Tsai MD (2002) Structure-based combinatorial protein engineering (SCOPE). J Mol Biol 321(4):677–691

11. Moore GL, Maranas CD (2000) Modeling DNA mutation and recombination for directed evolution experiments. J Theor Biol 205(3):483–503. doi:10.1006/jtbi.2000.2082

12. Moore GL, Maranas CD, Lutz S, Benkovic SJ (2001) Predicting crossover generation in DNA shuffling. Proc Natl Acad Sci U S A 98(6):3226–3231. doi:10.1073/pnas.051631498

13. Moore GL, Maranas CD (2002) eCodonOpt: a systematic computational framework for optimizing codon usage in directed evolution experiments. Nucleic Acids Res 30(11):2407–2416

14. He L, Friedman AM, Bailey-Kellogg C (2012) Algorithms for optimizing cross-overs in DNA shuffling. BMC Bioinformatics 13(Suppl 3):S3. doi:10.1186/1471-2105-13-s3-s3

Part II

DNA Synthesis, Assembly, and Cloning

Chapter 4

Simple Cloning by Prolonged Overlap Extension-PCR with Application to the Preparation of Large-Size Random Gene Mutagenesis Library in *Escherichia coli*

Chao Zhong, Chun You, Ping Wei, and Yi-Heng Percival Zhang

Abstract

We developed a simple method (simple cloning) for subcloning DNA fragments into any location of a targeted vector without the need of restriction enzyme, ligase, exonuclease, or recombinase in *Escherichia coli*. This technology can be applied to common *E. coli* hosts (e.g., DH5α, JM109, TOP10, BL21(DE3)). The protocol includes three steps: (1) generate DNA insert and linear vector backbone by regular high-fidelity PCR, where these two DNA fragments contain 3′ and 5′ overlapping termini; (2) generate DNA multimers based on these two DNA fragments by using prolonged overlap extension-PCR (POE-PCR) without primers added; and (3) transform POE-PCR product to competent *Escherichia coli* cells directly, yielding the desired plasmid. Simple cloning provides a new cloning method with great simplicity and flexibility. Furthermore, this new method can be modified for the preparation of a large-size mutant library for directed evolution in *E. coli*. Using this method, it is very easy to generate a mutant library with a size of more than 10^7 per 50 μL of the POE-PCR product within 1 day.

Key words Enzyme-free cloning, *Escherichia coli*, Prolonged overlap extension-PCR, Simple cloning, Directed evolution, High transformation efficiency

1 Introduction

Escherichia coli stains are widely used in the biotechnology industry and biological science studies. They are the most preferred model microorganisms for molecular cloning and recombinant protein expression, mainly due to the clear genetic background, fast growth rate under laboratory conditions, good transformation ability for hosting foreign DNA, and laboratory safety [1]. The most commonly used molecular cloning technology in *E. coli* is based on restriction enzymes that digest an inserted DNA fragment and vector and a DNA ligase that connects two fragments to yield the desired plasmid [2]. However, limited choices of restriction enzymes and their cutting sites, relatively low efficiencies in digestion and ligation, and possible self-ligation of the digested vector

Randall A. Hughes (ed.), *Synthetic DNA: Methods and Protocols*, Methods in Molecular Biology, vol. 1472,
DOI 10.1007/978-1-4939-6343-0_4, © Springer Science+Business Media New York 2017

may sometimes result in difficulties in obtaining positive colonies within a short time [3]. In addition, the use of restriction enzymes usually introduces the addition of several amino acids at the N- and C-termini of the target protein, and such addition could cause unexpected effects on the biochemical properties or expression levels of proteins [4].

To overcome such drawbacks in cloning methods based on restriction enzymes and ligase, several companies have developed recombinase-based cloning technologies, such as the Invitrogen Gateway cloning technology, Clonetech In-Fusion, BioCat Cold-Fusion, and Red/ET Recombination systems [5]. However, these recombinase-based cloning technologies heavily rely on specialized kits containing special vectors, enzymes, or hosts.

Restriction enzyme-based cloning methods are still the popular method to construct DNA mutant library for enzyme-directed evolution [6, 7]. The construction of a mutant library with reasonable size requires careful design (e.g., restriction enzymes and sequences of the targeted protein gene and vector) and a series of optimizations in fragment digestion, ligation, and transformation, which demands high skills and can be challenging for beginners [8].

Here we present a simple and easy cloning method based on the use of DNA multimers generated by prolonged overlap extension-PCR (POE-PCR) [9, 10]. This method has some differences from regular overlap extension PCR, for example (1) PCR primers are designed to be complementary for the amplification of a targeted vector and an insert gene, and (2) DNA multimers are generated by POE-PCR based on two PCR products featuring the overlap regions at the 5' and 3' ends without the presence of any primers. Such DNA multimers can be transformed into common laboratory *E. coli* hosts (e.g., DH5α, JM109, TOP10, BL21(DE3)) that are capable of cleaving assimilated DNA multimers into the circular plasmid, finally yielding a chimeric plasmid. By this new sequence-independent cloning method, the desired positive colonies can be obtained within 1 day even without validation of colony PCR before DNA sequencing.

In addition, a new protocol has been developed based on the use of the DNA multimers generated by POE-PCR to create a large-size library for enzyme-directed evolution in *E. coli* [11]. The DNA multimers can be digested by one restriction enzyme whose cutting site can be located anywhere on the vector backbone, yielding linear plasmid molecules. After self-ligation by DNA ligase, the circular plasmid is transformed to competent cells with very high transformation efficiencies, resulting in a large-size protein mutant library. In this method, labor-intensive optimizations in two restriction enzymes' digestion and ligation were not needed. As a result, a beginner can obtain a large-size mutant library of more than 10^7 cfu from 50 μL of the PCR product within 1 day.

2 Materials

2.1 Biological and Chemical Materials

1. Phusion DNA polymerase and Taq polymerase. Store at –20 °C (*see* **Note 1**).

2. 5× HF PCR buffer or 5× GC PCR buffer for PCR (provided with the Phusion polymerase), 10× Standard Taq Buffer (provided with the Taq polymerase). Store at –20 °C.

3. Deoxynucleotide solution mix (dNTP, 10 mM each). Store at –20 °C.

4. Oligonucleotide primers synthesized by Integrated DNA Technologies (Coralville, IA, USA) or other companies. Make the concentration of primers to 100 μM by adding appropriate amount of ultrapure water. Store them at –20 °C until used.

5. Plasmids and/or genomic DNA for PCR amplification template.

6. DNA Clean and Concentrator Kit from Zymo Research (Irvine, CA) or its equivalent.

7. Gel DNA recovery kit from Zymo Research or its equivalent.

8. Plasmid Miniprep isolation kit from Zymo Research or its equivalent.

9. NEB restriction enzymes or their equivalents.

10. Restriction enzyme buffer (provided with commercial restriction enzymes).

11. NEB Quick Ligation kit and its equivalent.

12. 0.8 % Agarose in 1× TAE buffer (40 mM Tris-acetate, 1 mM EDTA) with ethidium bromide.

13. Sterile SOC liquid medium: 0.5 % Yeast extract, 2 % tryptone, 10 mM NaCl, 2.5 mM KCl, 10 mM $MgCl_2$, 10 mM $MgSO_4$, 20 mM glucose. Autoclave the solution without glucose. Sterilize the glucose solution by passing it through a 0.2 μm filter. Mix two solutions together. SOC medium can be stored at room temperature and is stable for several years.

14. Lysogeny Broth (LB) medium: 1 % Bacto-tryptone, 0.5 % yeast extract, and 1 % NaCl in deionized water. For plates, 1.5 % agar is added.

2.2 Equipment

1. PCR thermocycler.

2. Agarose gel running system.

3. Nanodrop ND-1000 Spectrophotometer or equivalent.

4. Centrifuge, Thermo MicroCL 21R Series, or equivalent.

5. Gel Documentation System, Bio-Rad, or equivalent.

3 Methods

3.1 Primer Design

A pair of primers (IF/IR) is used to amplify the DNA fragment of insertion and the other pair of primers (VF/VR) is used to amplify the vector backbone (Fig. 1). VF, a 50 bp forward primer for vector linearization, contains the last 25 bp of 3′ terminal from the insert sequence and the first 25 bp of 5′ terminal from the vector sequence. IF, a 50 bp forward primer for amplifying the insertion, contains the last 25 bp of 3′ terminal from the vector sequence and the first 25 bp of 5′ terminal from the insert sequence (*see* **Note 2**). IF and VF are the reverse complementary sequences of VR and IR, respectively, and the melting temperatures (T_m) of IF and VR should be very similar, as well as VF and IR. These two melting temperatures should be designed to match with each other as closely as possible to decrease mis-hybridization.

3.2 Simple Cloning

Figure 2 represents the general scheme of simple cloning and modified simple cloning for mutant library construction. An example of the simple cloning method for subcloning of a DNA fragment encoding the UDP-glucose 4-epimerase gene (930 bp) into vector pET20b is outlined as follows (Fig. 3a):

1. Amplify the vector backbone with the VF and VR primer pair via PCR using a high-fidelity polymerase, such as Phusion DNA polymerase. The PCR reaction contains 200 μM dNTP mixtures, 0.5 μM of each primers, 0.05 ng/μL template DNA, 1× HF or GC buffer (*see* **Note 3**), and 0.02 U/μL Phusion DNA polymerase. The PCR program is 98 °C denaturation, 30 s; 30 cycles of 98 °C denaturation, 15 s; 55 °C annealing (*see* **Note 4**), 15 s; extension at 72 °C at 3 kb per minute for

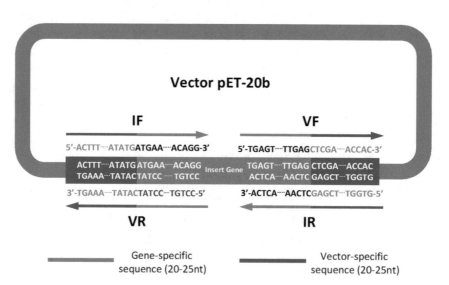

Fig. 1 Primers design for simple cloning that can insert one DNA fragment into any location within a plasmid

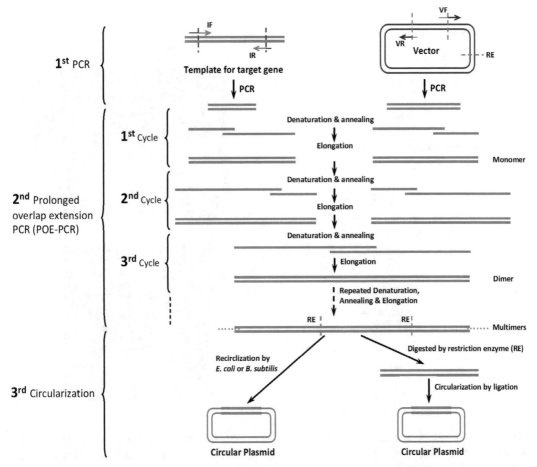

Fig. 2 Flow schemes of simple cloning by POE-PCR and generation of circular plasmid. First, the 3′ and 5′ overlapping insert and vector fragments are generated by standard PCR; for library construction, the mutant insert fragments are generated by error-prone PCR or DNA shuffling. Second, DNA multimers are formed in vitro by prolonged overlap extension-PCR. Third, *E. coli* strains can cleave DNA multimers to a circular plasmid, the desired chimeric plasmid; for library construction, the DNA multimers are digested by a restriction enzyme followed by ligation to yield the circular plasmids

the targeted fragment; followed by a 5-min extension at 72 °C. The quality of the PCR product can be checked by examining 2 μL of the product by 0.8 % agarose gel electrophoresis (Fig. 3b, lane 1).

2. Amplify the insert fragment with the IF and IR primer pair by PCR by using a high-fidelity DNA polymerase such as Phusion DNA polymerase. Its quality can be checked by examining 2 μL of the product by 0.8 % agarose gel electrophoresis (Fig. 3b, lane 2).

3. Clean up the two PCR products with a DNA Clean and Concentrator Kit or similar products (*see* **Note 5**).

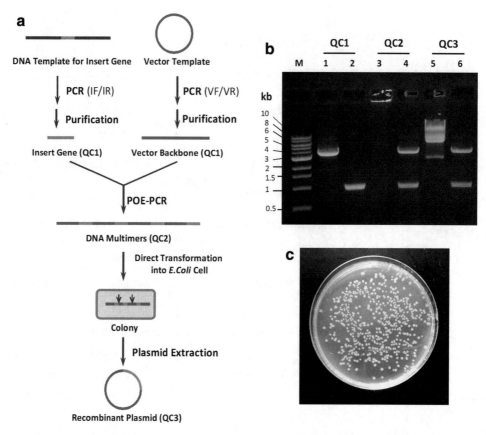

Fig. 3 (**a**) Overview of simple cloning and DNA assembly by POE-PCR. (**b**) Simple cloning for one insertion and vector. Lanes: *M*, DNA markers; *lane 1* PCR-linearized pET20b vector, *lane 2* PCR-linearized UDP-glucose 4-epimerase insert, *lane 3* DNA multimers generated by prolonged overlap extension-PCR, *lane 4* PCR products digested with NdeI and XhoI, *lane 5* a purified plasmid from a randomly selected *E. coli* colony, *lane 6* a purified plasmid digested with NdeI and XhoI; and M, 1 kb DNA ladder from NEB. (**c**) The transformants shown on the plate were the result of directly transforming the above reaction into *E. coli*

4. Determine the concentration of two purified DNA fragments with a Nanodrop ND-1000 Spectrophotometer or by estimating the concentration from the agarose gel by using DNA standards of known quantity.

5. For the generation of DNA multimers by POE-PCR, prepare the PCR solution as follows: 1× HF or GC buffer, 0.2 mM dNTP mixtures, 5 ng/μL vector backbone, equimolar amount of the insert DNA fragment (*see* **Note 6**), and 0.02 U/μL Phusion DNA polymerase in a total volume of 50 μL.

6. POE-PCR is conducted as follows: 98 °C denaturation, 30 s; 30 cycles of 98 °C denaturation, 15 s, 55 °C annealing 15 s, extension at 72 °C for 2 kb per minute based on the length of the resulting plasmid; and 10-min extension at 72 °C. Here the extension time was about 1.5-fold of the extension time of typical overlap extension-PCR.

7. The quality of the POE-PCR product can be examined by adding 2 μL of the product in 0.8% agarose gel (*see* **Note 7**). The DNA multimers are high-molecular-weight products so that they cannot migrate into the gel (Fig. 3b, lane 3) (*see* **Note 8**). Also, the quality of the POE-PCR product can be examined by restriction enzyme digestion, where the resulting digestion pattern should be the same result as if the desired plasmid was digested by the same enzyme(s) (Fig. 3b, lanes 4 and 6).

8. Transform the DNA multimers into *E. coli* cells as follows: Gently mix 2–5 μL of the POE-PCR product (*see* **Note 9**) with 100 μL competent *E. coli* cells in a 1.5 mL polypropylene tube. Place the tube on ice for 20 min, at 42 °C for 90 s, followed by on ice for 5 min. Add 1 mL of the SOC liquid medium into the tube; incubate the tube at 37 °C for 30 min. After centrifugation at $2500 \times g$ for 5 min, discard 1 mL of the supernatant. Resuspend the cell pellets with the remaining liquid, and then spread the cells on one Petri plate containing LB solid medium supplemented with appropriate antibiotic. Incubate the plate at 37 °C for 12–16 h or until the colonies could be easily be seen (Fig. 3c). Typical transformation efficiencies are ~ 1–3×10^4 per μg of the DNA multimer product by using homemade cells with a transformation efficiency of $\sim 1 \times 10^7$ per μg of plasmid. To verify successful cloning of the insert into the vector, colonies can be checked by colony PCR using primers IF/IR. In the example given, the 930 bp bands were obtained in the resulting PCR products for all the randomly picked colonies, indicating that almost all the transformants were positive for the cloned insert.

9. Pick one of the transformants from the plate and inoculate it into 3–5 mL of the LB medium supplemented with appropriate antibiotic and incubate at 37 °C for 10–12 h. Following growth, extract the plasmid by a Plasmid Miniprep isolation kit.

10. Check the plasmid (Fig. 3b, lane 5) and its restriction digestion product (Fig. 3b, lane 6) by 0.8% agarose gel electrophoresis.

11. If necessary, the plasmid can be sequenced for further validation.

3.3 Easy Preparation of a Large-Size Random Gene Mutagenesis Library

A detailed process for preparation of a large-size library for directed evolution in *E. coli* based on DNA multimers generated by POE-PCR is described as follows:

1. To demonstrate the preparation and cloning of a library of gene sequences by the POE-PCR method, a template plasmid containing the gene to be mutagenized must be constructed. As an example, a 706 bp DNA sequence encoding mCherry fluorescent protein was used as the parental gene, which was amplified with a pair of primers (IF_mcherry: TTAAC TTTAA

GAAGG AGATA TACAT ATGGT GAGCA AGGGC GAGGA GGATA; IR_mcherry: CAGTT CATTA TCTGC CCACA GCTTA TCAGA ACCTG GCTTG) using Phusion DNA polymerase. The linear vector backbone containing the gene of a carbohydrate-binding module (CBM) was amplified with a pair of primers (VF_mcherry: CAAGC CAGGT TCTGA TAAGC TGTGG GCAGA TAATG AACTG; VR_mcherry: TATCC TCCTC GCCCT GCTCC ACCAT ATGTA TATCT CCTTC TTAAA GTTAA) using the Phusion DNA polymerase. The insert fragment and vector backbone were assembled into DNA multimers by POE-PCR as described above. The DNA multimers were then transferred to *E. coli* cells, yielding the template plasmid pET20b-mcherry-cbm (Fig. 4a).

2. To generate a mutant library of DNA sequences, the template plasmid created in Subheading 3.3, **step 1**, can be mutagenized by error-prone PCR (epPCR). The mCherry fluorescent protein gene was amplified with the IF_mcherry and IR_mcherry primers using epPCR conditions as follows: 1× standard Taq buffer, 0.02 ng/μL template plasmid pET20b-mcherry-cbm, 0.2 mM dATP, 0.2 mM dGTP, 1 mM dCTP, 1 mM dTTP, 5 mM MgCl$_2$, 0.2 mM MnCl$_2$ (*see* **Note 10**), 0.05 U/μL standard Taq polymerase, 0.4 μM IF_cherry primer, and 0.4 μM IR_cherry primer in a total volume of 50 μL. The PCR was cycled as follows: 94 °C denaturation for 2 min, 13–16 cycles of 94 °C denaturation for 30 s, 60 °C annealing for 30 s, 68 °C extension for 45 s, and 68 °C extension for 5 min.

3. Clean up the PCR products of vector backbone and mutant insert fragment using a DNA Clean and Concentrator Kit or similar. Verify successful amplification of the DNA by examining 2 μL of the resulting products on a 0.8 % agarose gel (Fig. 4b, lane 1–2).

4. Determine the concentration of two purified DNA fragments with a Nanodrop Spectrophotometer (or similar) or estimate the concentration according to agarose gel electrophoresis.

5. Generate DNA multimers of the mutagenized library by POE-PCR as follows: 0.2 mM dNTP mixtures, 5 ng/μL vector backbone, equimolar amount of the insert DNA fragment, and 0.04 U/μL Phusion DNA polymerase in a total volume of 50 μL. The POE-PCR was cycled at 98 °C denaturation, 30 s; 30 cycles of 98 °C denaturation, 10 s; 60 °C annealing, 10 s; and extension at 72 °C at a rate of 2 kb/min based on the length of the resulting plasmid.

6. Examine the quality of the POE-PCR product by running 2 μL of the product on a 0.8 % agarose gel to check the formation of DNA multimers (Fig. 4b, lane 3). Additionally, a 2 μL aliquot of the PCR product can be digested by restriction enzymes to check the plasmid map with 0.8 % agarose gel electrophoresis (Fig. 4b, lane 4).

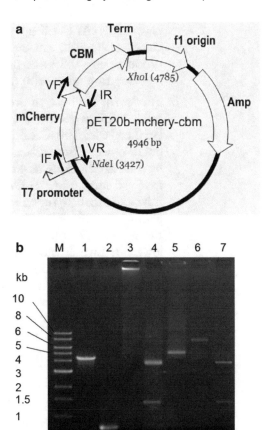

Fig. 4 (**a**) Map of the vector pET20b-mcherry-cbm. The *arrows* show the transcription directions for these genes. mcherry, wild-type mCherry-encoding sequence; cbm, family 17 carbohydrate-binding module-encoding sequence. IF, IR, VF, and VR denote the positions of the primers for PCR. (**b**) DNA analysis by agarose gel electrophoresis. *Lane M*, NEB 1 kb DNA ladder; *lane 1*, linear vector of pET20b containing cbm generated by regular PCR; *lane 2*, mcherry DNA generated by regular PCR; *lane 3*, DNA multimers generated by POE-PCR; *lane 4*, DNA multimers digested with Ndel and Xhol; *lane 5*, Xhol-digested DNA multimers; *lane 6*, circular plasmids after Xhol digestion followed by T4 ligation; *lane 7*, digested circular plasmids with Ndel and Xhol

7. Digest the POE-PCR product (DNA multimers) by a restriction enzyme digestion (*see* **Note 11**). The digestion conditions should be as follows: 1× restriction enzyme reaction buffer, 45 µL POE-PCR product, 0.2 mg/mL bovine serum albumin (BSA), and 0.2 U/µL restriction enzyme in a final volume of 200 µL. The reaction solution should be incubated at 37 °C (or the optimum temperature for the chosen restriction enzyme) for 2–3 h. The restriction-digested DNA multimers were applied to a 0.8 % agarose gel for electrophoresis (Fig. 4b, lane 5). Purify the linear plasmid DNAs in the targeted size with a Gel DNA recovery kit. Re-circularize the purified linear

plasmid DNAs (~1.5 µg) by ligation (*see* **Note 12**). The efficiency of ligation can be checked by examining 2 µL of the products on a 0.8% agarose gel (Fig. 4b, lane 6), or examined by restriction enzyme(s) digestion (Fig. 4b, lane 7).

8. Transform the ligation products (circular plasmid) into *E. coli* cells as follows: Gently mix 2–5 µL of the ligation product (~50 ng) with 100 µL of the competent *E. coli* cells in a 1.5 mL polypropylene tube. Place the tube on ice for 30 min, followed by thermal shocking at 42 °C for 90 s. Place the tube back on ice for 5 min. Add 1 mL of the SOC liquid medium into the tube and incubate the tube at 37 °C for 30 min. After centrifugation at $4000 \times g$ for 5 min, discard 1 mL of the supernatant. Resuspend the cell pellets with the remaining liquid or followed by further medium dilution, and then spread the cells on one Petri plate containing LB solid medium supplemented with appropriate antibiotic. Incubate the plate at 37 °C for 12–16 h or until colonies form (Fig. 5a). When competent cells with a transformation efficiency of 1×10^9 per µg of plasmid were used, the transformation of 2 µL of the ligation product could result in the colony number of up to 200,000. It means that at least 100–1000 times dilution is needed for obtaining 200–2000 colonies per dish.

9. Figure 5 shows typical results for the protein mutant library by this technology, where mCherry protein was used as an example. Approximately 70% of colonies were colorless (Fig. 5a), suggesting that most of the mutants were negative. Several fluorescent protein mutants exhibiting different colors were easily identified in Petri dish plates.

10. Pick some of the colonies from the transformation plate and inoculate into 3–5 mL of the LB medium supplemented with appropriate antibiotic and incubate at 37 °C for 10–12 h. Extract plasmids by Plasmid Miniprep isolation kit. The plasmids can be sequenced for further analysis. For example, four purified mCherry protein mutants exhibited different colors under natural visible lights and ultraviolet (UV) excitation (Fig. 5b, c).

4 Notes

1. To avoid possible mutations during the two-round PCR process, high-fidelity DNA polymerase must be used. High-fidelity DNA polymerases with a feature of long DNA fragment amplification are preferred for DNA assembly.

2. We usually use the overlap region of 25 bp, which means that the primers will be 50 bp. Based on our experience, the overlap region should be at least ~20 bp for good performance of

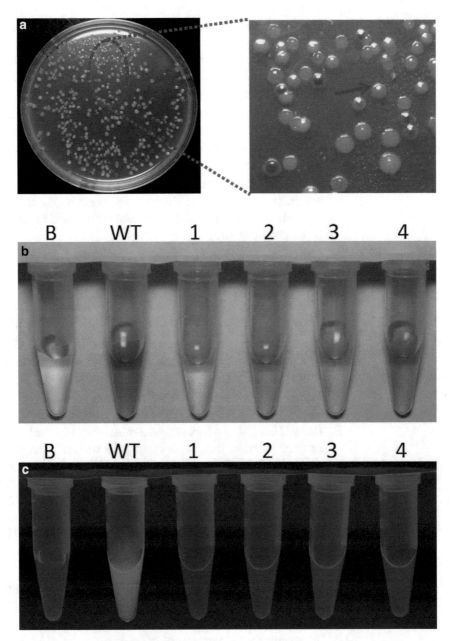

Fig. 5 Screening of mCherry fluorescence protein mutants expressed in *E. coli* BL21(DE3) on a Petri dish plate (**a**), where colonies containing wild-type or neutral mutants are *red*, a *yellow* colony represents a mutant with a new fluorescent color, and most *white* colonies reflect new type of mutant. (**b** and **c**) Purified fluorescent proteins with the same concentrations under natural visible light (**b**) and under UV excitation (**c**). *B* blank buffer, *WT* wild-type mCherry fluorescent protein; 1–4, mCherry mutants 1, 2, 3, and 4

the overlap extension process. The overlap region could be longer, but longer primer may result in a higher possibility to get mutations in the synthesized primers and the unit price for primers will be much higher when they exceed 60 bp.

3. It is recommended to first try the PCR with the HF buffer. If the PCR amplification in the HF buffer failed, then the GC buffer can be used because it can improve the performance of the Phusion DNA polymerase on templates that are long and GC rich or have complex secondary structures.

4. The annealing temperature can be determined by T_m calculator which is available in NEB website. If PCR amplification failed, optimize the annealing temperature by using gradient temperature PCR.

5. Sometimes the PCR product can contain some nonspecific bands. If this is the case, the targeted band based on its migration rate can be cut from the gel and be purified by using a Gel DNA recovery kit.

6. The amount of insert fragment added in the tube can be calculated based on the length of insertion. Here, the insertion length is 0.9 kb, the vector length is 3.4 kb, and the final concentration of vector is 5 ng/μL. So the final concentration of equimolar insert with the vector should be $5 \times 0.9/3.4 = 1.3$ ng/μL.

7. If no DNA multimers were generated by POE-PCR, PCR conditions can be optimized by (a) decreasing the annealing temperature, (b) increasing the template amount, (c) increasing the extension time in the POE-PCR, and (d) adding PCR-enhancing reagents, such as betaine or DMSO.

8. The POE-PCR product can be a quite viscous solution and can be used to transform competent cells directly. Do not try to clean the POE-PCR product with a DNA cleaning kit. The DNA multimers may be stored at 4 °C for several days for future transformation. Do not freeze the POE-PCR product since it can result in precipitation of the multimers. It is common to see some high-molecular-weight DNA above 10 kb on the agarose gel instead of DNA multimers; these are intermediates generated by POE-PCR.

9. Do not add too much POE-PCR product to the competent cells for transformation, since the high-salt PCR solution could decrease the transformation efficiency [12].

10. Increasing the concentration of Mn^{2+} up to 0.5 mM, increasing the concentration of Mg^{2+} up to 10 mM, and adding unequal amounts of the four dNTPs can increase the mutation rate.

11. The cutting site of restriction enzyme can be located anywhere on the desired plasmid, and can cut once in the desired plasmid sequence. It is recommended that the cutting site be located in the vector backbone, because a restriction site chosen within the inserted mutant library might not be available after mutagenesis. If there is not an appropriate cutting site in the vector backbone, the primers can be designed to contain a unique

restriction enzyme cutting site. High-affinity restriction enzyme featuring decreased star activity, such as BamH I-HF, EcoR I-HF, and Hind III-HF, is highly recommended.

12. In the classic two-fragment ligation protocol, the optimization of the ratio between two DNA fragments is vital to achieve high transformation efficiency. However, lab-intensive optimization was not needed because of one-fragment ligation. It is apparent that the efficiency of one-fragment circularization is much higher than two-fragment ligation.

Acknowledgement

This work could not be finished without the support of the Nanjing Tech University and Virginia Tech. In addition, funding to YPZ for this work was provided in part by DOE EERE award (DE-EE0006968) and by the Virginia Agricultural Experiment Station and the Hatch Program of the National Institute of Food and Agriculture, US Department of Agriculture.

References

1. Moxon ER, Higgins CF (1997) *E. coli* gene sequence - a blueprint for life. Nature 389:120–121

2. Sambrook J, Russell DW (2001) Molecular cloning: a laboratory manual. Cold Spring Harbor Laboratory, New York

3. Lund AH, Duch M, Pedersen FS (1996) Increased cloning efficiency by temperature-cycle ligation. Nucleic Acids Res 24:800–801

4. Young TS, Schultz PG (2010) Beyond the canonical 20 amino acids: expanding the genetic lexicon. J Biol Chem 285:11039–11044

5. Li CA, Evans RM (1997) Ligation independent cloning irrespective of restriction site compatibility. Nucleic Acids Res 25:4165–4166

6. Gillam EMJ, Copp JN, Ackerley DF et al (2014) Directed evolution library creation: methods and protocols, 2nd edn. Springer, New York

7. Abou-Nader M, Benedik MJ (2010) Rapid generation of random mutant libraries. Bioeng Bugs 1:337–340

8. Pai JC, Entzminger KC, Maynard JA (2012) Restriction enzyme-free construction of random gene mutagenesis libraries in *Escherichia coli*. Anal Biochem 421:640–648

9. You C, Zhang X-Z, Zhang YHP (2012) Simple cloning via direct transformation of PCR product (DNA Multimer) to *Escherichia coli* and *Bacillus subtilis*. Appl Environ Microbiol 78:1593–1595

10. Zhang X-Z, Zhang YHP (2011) Simple, fast and high-efficiency transformation system for directed evolution of cellulase in *Bacillus subtilis*. Microb Biotechnol 4:98–105

11. You C, Zhang YHP (2012) Easy preparation of a large-size random gene mutagenesis library in *Escherichia coli*. Anal Biochem 428:7–12

12. Shafikhani S, Siegel RA, Ferrari E et al (1997) Generation of large libraries of random mutants in *Bacillus subtilis* by PCR-based plasmid multimerization. Biotechniques 23:304–310

Chapter 5

SpeedyGenes: Exploiting an Improved Gene Synthesis Method for the Efficient Production of Synthetic Protein Libraries for Directed Evolution

Andrew Currin, Neil Swainston, Philip J. Day, and Douglas B. Kell

Abstract

Gene synthesis is a fundamental technology underpinning much research in the life sciences. In particular, synthetic biology and biotechnology utilize gene synthesis to assemble any desired DNA sequence, which can then be incorporated into novel parts and pathways. Here, we describe SpeedyGenes, a gene synthesis method that can assemble DNA sequences with greater fidelity (fewer errors) than existing methods, but that can also be used to encode extensive, statistically designed sequence variation at any position in the sequence to create diverse (but accurate) variant libraries. We summarize the integrated use of GeneGenie to design DNA and oligonucleotide sequences, followed by the procedure for assembling these accurately and efficiently using SpeedyGenes.

Key words Directed evolution, Error correction, Gene synthesis, Protein libraries, Synthetic biology

1 Introduction

Gene synthesis is an important driving force behind the developing disciplines of synthetic biology and biotechnology. Reducing cost and increased throughput have enabled the emergence of synthetic biology, where any desired DNA sequence can be synthesized and then assembled into pathways and genomes. However, this technology is hindered by the frequency at which errors occur in the synthesized sequence, an issue that generally arises from the oligonucleotide building blocks from which it is assembled. Consequently, there is a strong demand for improvements in these methodologies to further increase the accuracy and efficiency of this process. In addition, an important requirement of biotechnology and synthetic biology is the ability to encode mutations to create variant libraries for screening of novel or altered functions. In this chapter we outline SpeedyGenes [1], an improved gene synthesis method that can assemble DNA with a greater accuracy

Randall A. Hughes (ed.), *Synthetic DNA: Methods and Protocols*, Methods in Molecular Biology, vol. 1472,
DOI 10.1007/978-1-4939-6343-0_5, © Springer Science+Business Media New York 2017

(fewer errors) than existing methods, but can also be extended to generate stable variant libraries *de novo* using mixed base codons.

Most enzymes have a rather modest catalytic activity [2], primarily due to the fact that natural evolution often did not have the need to select for significantly greater activity within its biological context [3, 4]. However, many biotechnology applications require the heterologous expression of proteins and pathways [5], and these must undergo further selection to optimize the system for its new objective(s) [6]. This has led to the development of "directed protein evolution" (e.g., [4, 7–9]), an iterative process of mutagenesis and selection [10] (Fig. 1), which selects for one or more fitnesses (fitness functions) that are of interest not to the organism but to the human experimenter. Such fitness or objective functions for enzymes often include substrate specificity, stereoselectivity, k_{cat}, and thermostability [4], albeit the "first rule" of directed evolution has been said to be that "you get what you select for (even if you did not mean to)."

Classically, protein diversity could be generated at the DNA level using random mutagenesis methods, primarily error-prone

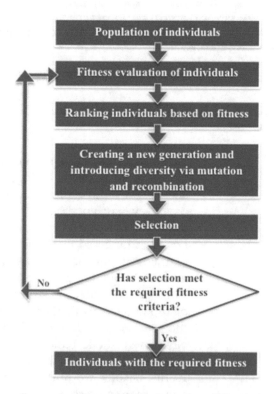

Fig. 1 The overall procedure for an evolutionary system. At the start, an individual protein is selected and assessed for its fitness (i.e., its activity). Genetic diversity then creates a library of variants, from which improved individuals are selected. This cycle is repeated until the individual fulfils the desired fitness criteria

PCR (epPCR, [11]) or "DNA shuffling" (the equivalent of recombination [12]). However, a fundamental problem is the simply vast extent of the search space of possible proteins [10, 13, 14], 20^{300} or $\sim10^{390}$ for an approximately average-sized protein of 300 amino acids. Purely random changes in sequence simply affect a local search, and substantial random mutations (that might widen the search) lead to the production of stop codons (3 per 64 residues) and premature truncation [15]. Additionally, epPCR is also limited by considerable bias towards transition mutations and also these single-base mutations cannot encode all possible amino acids [16].

In contrast, the advent of large-scale *synthetic* DNA methods, (even at the whole-genome level [17]), means that it is now possible to target specific residues with specific mutations, which thereby circumvents many of the above problems and permits a massively improved means to navigate these very large search spaces [4]. We have developed both computational (GeneGenie [18]) and experimental (SpeedyGenes [1]) strategies for performing this. Our novel experimental workflow simultaneously corrects the sequence errors in the full sequence while allowing the incorporation of any desired variation at precise residues (and at potentially enormous rates). The results of a given generation can then be used to design (again statistically) the kinds of sequence variation one might desire for subsequent generations (as we have done for aptamers [19]). It is this "eyes open" strategy that permits the intelligent navigation of (even highly epistatic) protein search spaces [4].

The purpose of this chapter is thus to provide a 'hands-on' guide to the use of GeneGenie and SpeedyGenes, both for efficient gene synthesis and experimental directed evolution studies.

2 Materials

1. High-fidelity DNA polymerase, preferably hot start.
2. 2 mM dNTP mix.
3. DNase-free high-purity water.
4. DNA oligonucleotides.
5. Surveyor endonuclease kit (Integrated DNA Technologies).
6. Thermal cycler.
7. DNA gel or capillary electrophoresis equipment.
8. Nanodrop (Thermo Scientific) or other spectrophotometer.
9. Set of pipettes.
10. PCR tubes.
11. Microcentrifuge tubes.
12. DNA purification kits, including PCR cleanup and gel extraction kits.

3   Methods

3.1   Design of DNA Oligonucleotides

The online tool GeneGenie (http://www.gene-genie.org) [18] has been created to facilitate the design of oligonucleotides for assembly using the SpeedyGenes method. At the outset of the project it is advised to plan the full experimental cloning approach, including the target plasmid and cloning strategy. Once these have been defined, the 5′ and 3′ sequences required for downstream cloning can be inputted into GeneGenie to be included in the optimised oligomer design.

1. Input the desired amino acid sequence into GeneGenie, together with the 5′ and 3′ DNA sequences required for downstream applications (Fig. 2, *see* **Notes 1** and **2**).

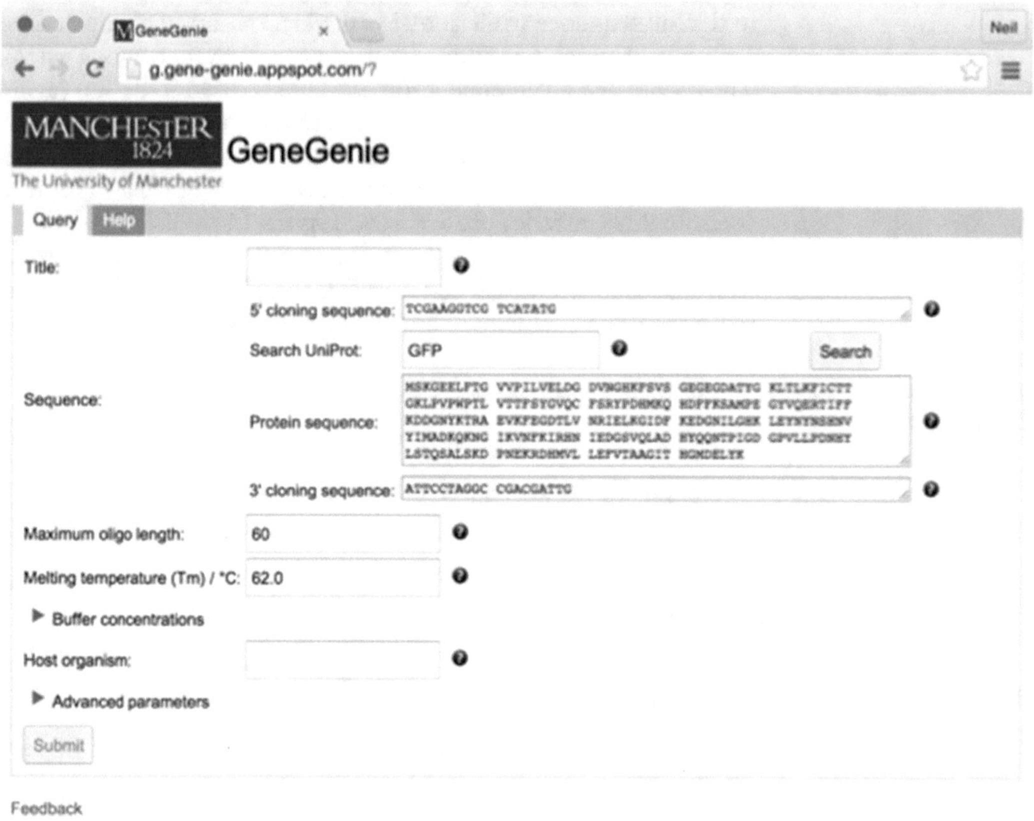

Fig. 2 The GeneGenie query page, allowing specification of the target protein sequence, 5′ and 3′ cloning sequences, maximum oligomer length, target melting temperature, and host organism for expression

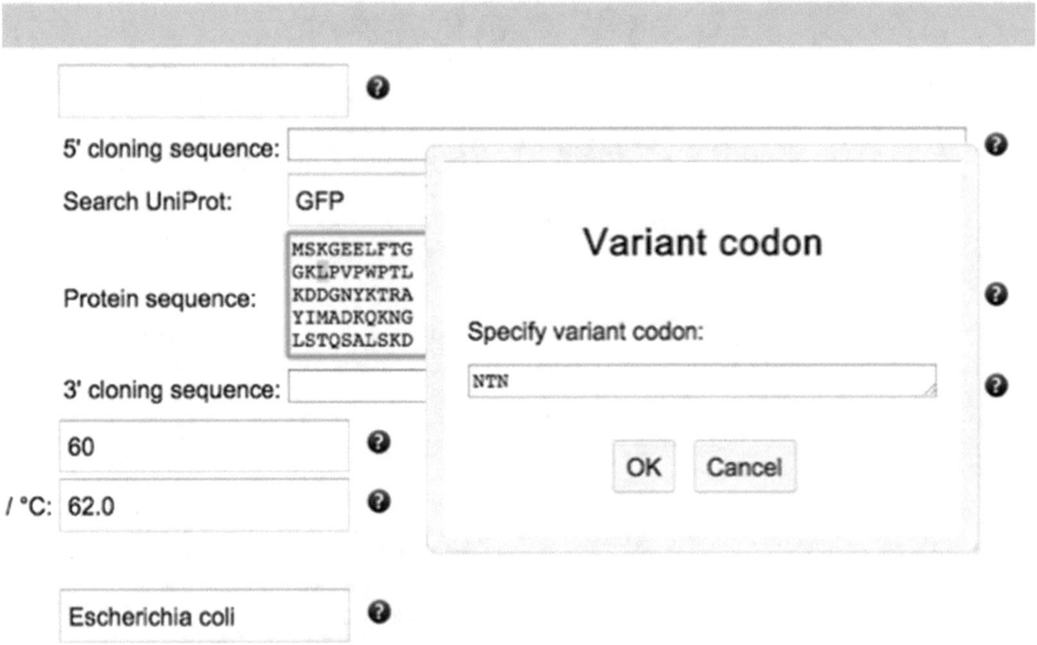

5' cloning sequence: ❓

Search UniProt: GFP

Variant codon

Protein sequence:
MSKGEELFTG
GKLPVPWPTL
KDDGNYKTRA
YIMADKQKNG
LSTQSALSKD

Specify variant codon:

3' cloning sequence: NTN

60 ❓

/ °C: 62.0 ❓

OK   Cancel

Escherichia coli ❓

Fig. 3 The GeneGenie query page, showing specification of the variant codon NTN at a specific position, introducing variability at this site and ultimately generating variant libraries

2. Set the design parameters, including desired melting temperature for oligonucleotide annealing and target organism for expression (*see* **Note 3**).

3. Mixed base codons can also be inputted at this stage in the design of variant libraries for directed evolution (Fig. 3, *see* **Note 4**).

3.2 Assembly of Non-variant Sequences

3.2.1 Intermediate Block Synthesis

For gene sequences of <600 bp it is possible to assemble these in one PCR; however for sequences >600 bp it is required to perform synthesis of multiple intermediate blocks in parallel (Fig. 4, *see* **Notes 5** and **6**).

1. Reconstitute the oligonucleotides to 100 μM in high-purity DNase-free water (*see* **Note 7**).

2. Create a 10 μM stock for each of the flanking oligonucleotides to be used as PCR primers for each of the intermediate blocks (e.g., for a block containing six oligonucleotides, numbers 1 and 6 are the flanking primers).

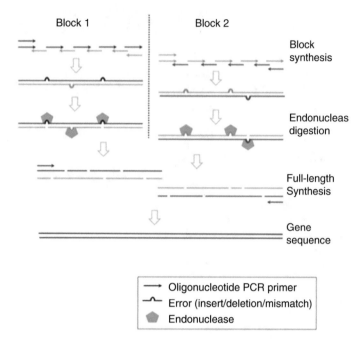

Fig. 4 The SpeedyGenes workflow for non-variant sequences. Genes are first assembled from DNA oligonucleotides into intermediate blocks (an example of two blocks is shown) using overlap-extension PCR (OE-PCR). These blocks then undergo incubation with the mismatch endonuclease Surveyor to cleave sequence errors. These digested products are then pooled together and used as the template for a second OE-PCR, which assembles the full-length, error-corrected sequence

3. To create the template, pool the remaining oligonucleotides (e.g., numbers 2–5) into a 600 nM mixture. This is a 1/166 dilution (from the 100 μM stock) for each oligonucleotide used in the assembly reaction.

4. Set up the PCR as follows (*see* **Notes 8** and **9**):

	Volume
600 nM Oligonucleotide mix template	2.5 μL
10 μM Forward primer	3 μL
10 μM Reverse primer	3 μL
2 mM dNTPs	5 μL
DNA polymerase buffer	As specified
High-fidelity DNA polymerase (hot start)	As specified
DNase-free water	Up to 50 μL

5. Carry out the PCR using a thermal cycler using the following settings:

	Temperature (°C)	Time (s)
Initial denaturation	98	120
35 cycles	98	10
	60 (or other T_m)	20
	72	20
Hold	4–10	

6. Purify the PCR products using a DNA purification kit following the manufacturer's instructions. Elute the DNA in 20 μL elution buffer.

7. Analyze the purified products using electrophoresis and measure the concentration using a spectrophotometer (*see* **Notes 10** and **11**).

3.2.2 Endonuclease Digestion for Error Correction

1. Dilute each purified intermediate block to 100 ng/μL in 1× DNA polymerase reaction buffer (*see* **Note 12**), in a total volume of 10 μL.

2. Perform the denaturation and slow hybridization to create mismatches:

	Temperature	Ramp rate (°C/s)	Time
Initial denaturation	95		2 min
Slow hybridization	85 °C	2	1 min
	Lowered in 10 °C intervals down to 25 °C	0.3	1 min at every 10 °C interval
Hold	4 °C		

3. Create the endonuclease enzyme mix (*see* **Note 13**).

	Volume
Surveyor endonuclease	2 μL
Surveyor enhancer	1 μL
1× DNA polymerase buffer	As specified
DNase-free water	Up to 5 μL

4. Combine 5 μL of the hybridized DNA with 5 μL of enzyme mix and gently mix.

5. Incubate at 42 °C on a thermocycler or heat block for 2 h.

6. Purify the digest products using a DNA purification kit, eluting with 10–20 μL elution buffer (*see* **Note 14**).

1. To create the PCR template, add 1 µL of each of the purified block digests together.

2. For PCR primers, use the two outermost oligonucleotides in the sequence.

3. Set up the PCR reaction as follows:

	Volume
Template	2 µL
10 µM Forward primer	3 µL
10 µM Reverse primer	3 µL
2 mM dNTPs	5 µL
DNA polymerase buffer	As specified
High-fidelity DNA polymerase (hot start)	As specified
DNase-free water	Up to 50 µL

4. Run the PCR using the following cycle (*see* **Note 15**):

	Temperature (°C)	Time (s)
Initial denaturation	98	120
35 cycles	98	10
	60 (or other T_m)	20
	72	40 (or longer as required)
Hold	4–10	

5. Analyze the PCR products using agarose gel electrophoresis (*see* **Note 11**).

3.3 Assembly of Variant Libraries

The three-step procedure of (1) block synthesis, (2) endonuclease digestion, and (3) full-length assembly is the same for the synthesis of variant and non-variant sequences. However, when oligonucleotides containing mixed base codons (here termed variant oligonucleotides) are to be used to create variant libraries, the block synthesis and full-length PCR steps are modified (Fig. 5). As such, the protocol in Subheading 3.2 should be carried out using the following alternative steps.

Subheading 3.2.1:

Alternative step 3. To create the template for the block synthesis, pool the desired oligonucleotides (including the variant oligonucleotides) into the 600 nM mixture.

Subheading 3.2.3:

Alternative step 3. Set up the PCR including the "spiked-in" variant oligonucleotides:

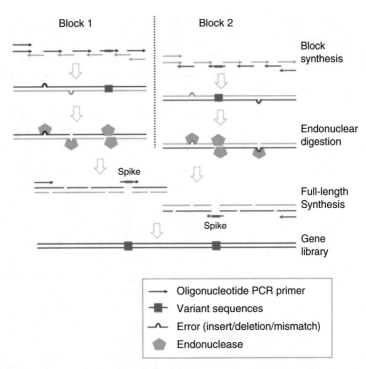

Fig. 5 The SpeedyGenes method for synthesis of variant libraries. Variant oligo-nucleotides are used for the intermediate block synthesis. These mixed base sequences are heavily digested by the Surveyor nuclease. Consequently, the same variant oligonucleotides are "spiked" into the final OE-PCR step to assemble the full-length variant sequence

	Volume
Template	2 μL
10 μM Forward primer	3 μL
10 μM Reverse primer	3 μL
0.1 μM Variant oligonucleotide(s)	3 μL
2 mM dNTPs	5 μL
DNA polymerase buffer	As specified
High-fidelity DNA polymerase (hot start)	As specified
DNase-free water	Up to 50 μL

Subheading 3.2.3:
Carry out the PCR as in Subheading 3.2.3, **step 4**.

3.4 Downstream Cloning and E. coli Transformation

The SpeedyGenes protocol has been developed using the In-Fusion cloning system (Clontech) to ligate into a linearized expression vector, however any cloning procedure can be used after the above procedures. Here, we outline our current procedure as an example workflow.

1. Run the SpeedyGenes PCR products on an agarose electro-phoresis gel and purify the full-length product (gene) using a gel extraction purification kit.

2. Ligate the gene into a linearized plasmid using the In-Fusion cloning kit, following the manufacturer's protocol.

3. Transform the ligation product into high-efficiency *E. coli* competent cells, purify the plasmid, and verify the correct sequences by DNA sequencing. For screening purposes, syn-thesized genes can be assayed directly from the transformation culture without the need for further sequence verification (Figs. 6, 7, and 8).

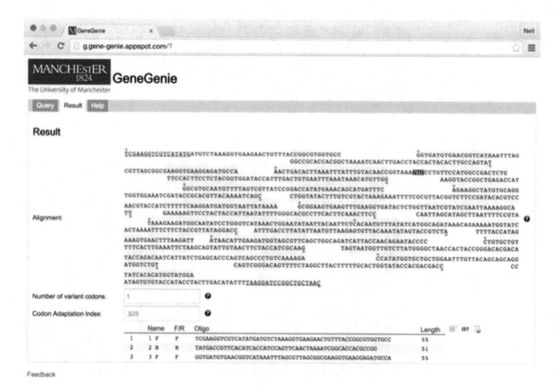

Fig. 6 A GeneGenie result page, showing the optimized oligomer design in terms of its alignment and list of oligo-mers to synthesise or purchase. 5′ and 3′ cloning sequences are underlined in the alignment, with variant codons highlighted in *green*. Other statistics, including those relating to optimized codon usage, are also displayed

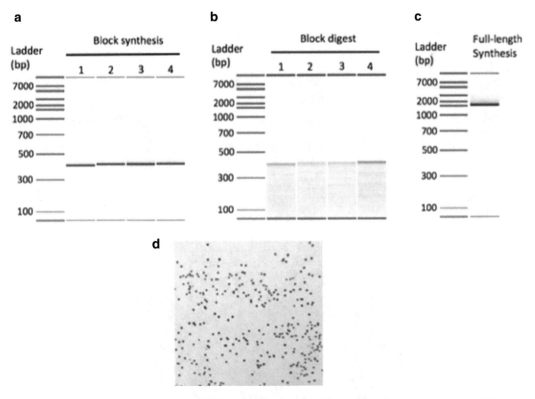

Fig. 7 Synthesis of a monoamine oxidase (MAO-N) and direct functional assay for catalytic activity. DNA fragments are analyzed using capillary electrophoresis. (**a**) The 1518 bp sequence was assembled using four intermediate blocks (labeled *1–4*), followed by (**b**) mismatch endonuclease digestion of the blocks. (**c**) Pooling of these digest products and assembly into the full MAO-N sequence by OE-PCR. (**d**) Direct ligation and expression of this gene in *E. coli* showed 76 % clones with full catalytic activity (and correct DNA sequence)

3.5 Concluding Remarks

The basis for the directed evolution of proteins lies in the ability to create and assay variant sequences for improved properties. Classical methods were more or less entirely empirical (random), but synthetic biology facilitates the means to create (statistically) precise variant DNA sequences *at any residue*. This permits the exploitation of (theoretically desirable [20]) high mutation rates without the potential creation of stop codons. However, DNA synthesis is itself prone to errors and standard error correction procedures might simply remove the diversity that one is seeking to create! SpeedyGenes [1, 4] circumvents this by separating the error-correction and diversity-introducing steps, with optimization controlled by the GeneGenie [18] software. In contrast to methods such as ProSAR [21], this permits the exploration and exploitation even of epistatic interactions, and hence the intelligent navigation [4] of the very large search spaces involved.

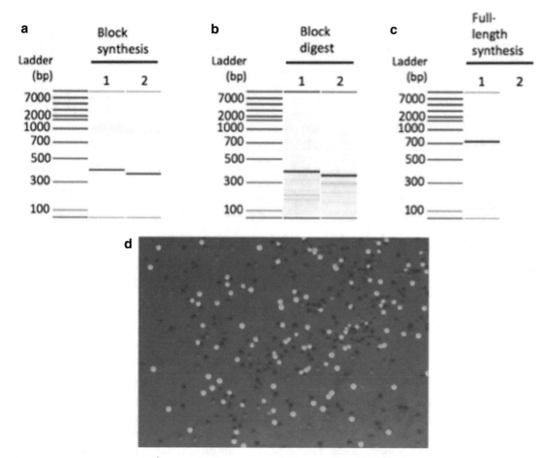

Fig. 8 Synthesis of controlled variant libraries of enhanced green fluorescent protein (EGFP). Residues 66 and 145 were mutated in a reduced library using mixed base codons, mutating these codons to encode Y/H and Y/F, respectively. The variant oligonucleotides encoding these mutations (6 and 12) were (**a**) assembled into the intermediate blocks then (**b**) subject to endonuclease digestion. (**c**) Variant oligonucleotides were then "spiked in" for the final OE-PCR step. (**d**) Expression of this library in *E. coli* identified both *green* and *blue* variants when analyzed under UV light

4   Notes

1. It is strongly advised to input the additional 5′ and 3′ sequences required for cloning into the initial GeneGenie designs. This will enable GeneGenie to include these sequences in its calculations to maximize the efficiency of the PCR assembly. If these sequences are not included at this design stage then it is possible that they may anneal in an incorrect position in the sequence, thus reducing the efficiency of the assembly. Incorporating 5′ and 3′ sequences optimizes the design of

oligomers encoding *both* the cloning sequences and the gene simultaneously.

2. Check that the 5′ and 3′ sequences include the required sequences for any downstream procedures. These commonly include (1) adding a start codon; (2) adding a stop codon; and (3) correction of the reading frame if using restriction endonucleases.

3. The length of oligonucleotides is often defined by the preferred supplier and synthesis scale required, while the melting temperature (T_m) is determined by the annealing temperature at which the PCR assembly will be performed. If the methodology does not yield good results, redesigning the gene using a higher T_m could resolve the issue.

4. If the design is to include mixed base codons for variant libraries, these should best be specified in the initial designs. When these are specified, GeneGenie will endeavor to design the oligonucleotides such that their positions do not fall within the overlap regions of the construct (enabling them to be mutated using a single oligonucleotide).

5. Intermediate blocks <600 bp can be reliably assembled using oligonucleotides. Synthesizing sequences >600 bp, or containing >12 oligonucleotides, often do not assemble with high efficiency. For example, for the 747 bp sequence for EGFP, this was separated into two blocks for efficient assembly.

6. For each intermediate block, the oligonucleotides at the outer 5′ and 3′ ends are used as PCR primers. It is therefore important that each block contains an equal number of oligonucleotides. For example, in a block containing six oligonucleotides, oligonucleotide 1 is the forward primer and 6 is the reverse primer.

7. This protocol has been developed using DNA oligonucleotides with a standard desalting purification. Other purifications, like HPLC, can be used but are not required. However, it is recommended that the oligonucleotides are of high quality with mass spectrometry analysis for quality control (Tables 1 and 2).

8. Use of a high-fidelity DNA polymerase is required for the protocol. During the final OE-PCR step (where the products from the endonuclease digest are assembled into the full-length sequence) the strong proofreading ability of this polymerase is crucial for the removal of the erroneous sequence for successful error correction. In addition, a high-fidelity polymerase will also minimize the introduction of new erroneous sequences during the PCR cycling steps. We routinely use the Q5 hot start high-fidelity polymerase (New England Biolabs).

Table 1
The IUPAC code [22] for mixed DNA bases

Symbol	Nucleotide base
G	G
A	A
T	T
C	C
R	G, A
Y	T, C
M	A, C
K	G, T
S	G, C
W	A, T
H	A, C, T
B	G, T, C
V	G, C, A
D	G, A, T
N	G, A, T, C

Table 2
An example of the mixed base codons that can be used for generating controlled genetic diversity

Degenerate codon	Mixed base sequence	Encoded codons	Stop codons	Encoded amino acids	Properties
NNN	(A, T, G, C) (A, T, G, C) (A, T, G, C)	64	TAA, TAG, TGA	All	Fully randomized codon
NNK	(A, T, G, C) (A, T, G, C) (G, T)	32		All	All 20 amino acids
NDT	(A, T, G, C) (A, T, G) T	12	No	Phe, Leu, Ile, Val, Tyr, His, Asn, Asp, Cys, Arg, Ser, Gly	Mixture of polar, nonpolar, positive, and negative charge (Reetz 2008)
NTN	(A, T, G, C) T (A, T, G, C)	16	No	Met, Phe, Leu, Ile, Val	Nonpolar residues

The number of possible codons, inclusion of stop codons, and the amino acids they encode are also highlighted

9. Use of a hot start DNA polymerase is also recommended to prevent undesired polymerization of the oligonucleotide template prior to PCR assembly. If using a non-hot start polymerase, then the reactions should be set up on ice and transferred directly to a preheated PCR machine at the start of the protocol.

10. When designing the thermal cycling protocols it is important to check the manufacturer's instructions for the DNA polymerase used. Importantly, this will recommend particular reaction conditions or cycling temperatures that should be used.

11. The thermal cycling conditions have a significant impact over the quality of the PCR products created. Hence, if nonspecific bands are detected then optimization of the annealing temperature, annealing time, and elongation time should be attempted.

12. A concentration of 70–100 ng/µL is desirable for each block for the endonuclease digestion. Lower concentrations can be used successfully, but it is desirable to use roughly equal concentrations of fragments in the final PCR assembly.

13. Due to the viscosity of the enzyme mix, it is recommended to create a larger stock mixture sufficient for all the digest reactions.

14. It is preferable to elute in a low volume at this step to maximize the DNA concentration.

15. Depending on the size of the sequence to be assembled it may be necessary to increase the extension time. Refer to the manufacturer's instructions for the recommended extension times for the DNA polymerase used.

Acknowledgements

We thank the Biotechnology and Biological Sciences Research Council for financial support (grant BB/M017702/1); Prof Nick Turner, Dr. Ian Rowles, and Dr. Timothy Eyes for useful discussions; and Mrs. Hannah Currin for preparation of figures. This is a contribution from the Manchester Centre for Synthetic Biology of Fine and Speciality Chemicals (SYNBIOCHEM).

References

1. Currin A, Swainston N, Day PJ, Kell DB (2014) SpeedyGenes: an improved gene synthesis method for the efficient production of error-corrected, synthetic protein libraries for directed evolution. Protein Eng Des Sel 27:273–280. doi:10.1093/protein/gzu029

2. Bar-Even A, Noor E, Savir Y, Liebermeister W, Davidi D, Tawfik DS, Milo R (2011) The moderately efficient enzyme: evolutionary and physicochemical trends shaping enzyme parameters. Biochemistry 50(21):4402–4410

3. Kacser H, Burns JA (1981) The molecular basis of dominance. Genetics 97:639–666

4. Currin A, Swainston N, Day PJ, Kell DB (2015) Synthetic biology for the directed evolution of protein biocatalysts: navigating sequence space intelligently. Chem Soc Rev 44(5):1172–1239. doi:10.1039/c1034cs00351a

5. Kell DB, Westerhoff HV (1986) Metabolic control theory: its role in microbiology and biotechnology. FEMS Microbiol Rev 39:305–320

6. Mendes P, Kell DB (1998) Non-linear optimization of biochemical pathways: applications to metabolic engineering and parameter estimation. Bioinformatics 14:869–883

7. Arnold FH, Volkov AA (1999) Directed evolution of biocatalysts. Curr Opin Chem Biol 3(1):54–59

8. Voigt CA, Kauffman S, Wang ZG (2001) Rational evolutionary design: the theory of *in vitro* protein evolution. Adv Protein Chem 55:79–160

9. Turner NJ (2009) Directed evolution drives the next generation of biocatalysts. Nat Chem Biol 5(8):567–573

10. Kell DB, Lurie-Luke E (2015) The virtue of innovation: innovation through the lenses of biological evolution. J R Soc Interface 12(2):20141183. doi:10.1098/rsif.2014.1183

11. McCullum EO, Williams BA, Zhang J, Chaput JC (2010) Random mutagenesis by error-prone PCR. Methods Mol Biol 634:103–109. doi:10.1007/978-1-60761-652-8_7

12. Stemmer WPC (1994) Rapid evolution of a protein *in vivo* by DNA shuffling. Nature 370:389–391

13. Reetz MT, Kahakeaw D, Lohmer R (2008) Addressing the numbers problem in directed evolution. Chembiochem 9(11):1797–1804

14. Kell DB (2012) Scientific discovery as a combinatorial optimisation problem: how best to navigate the landscape of possible experiments? Bioessays 34(3):236–244

15. Pritchard L, Corne DW, Kell DB, Rowland JJ, Winson MK (2004) A general model of error-prone PCR. J Theor Biol 234(4):497–509

16. Zhao J, Kardashliev T, Joelle Ruff A, Bocola M, Schwaneberg U (2014) Lessons from diversity of directed evolution experiments by an analysis of 3,000 mutations. Biotechnol Bioeng 111:2380–2389. doi:10.1002/bit.25302

17. Gibson DG, Benders GA, Andrews-Pfannkoch C, Denisova EA, Baden-Tillson H, Zaveri J, Stockwell TB, Brownley A, Thomas DW, Algire MA, Merryman C, Young L, Noskov VN, Glass JI, Venter JC, Hutchison CA III, Smith HO (2008) Complete chemical synthesis, assembly, and cloning of a *Mycoplasma genitalium* genome. Science 319(5867):1215–1220

18. Swainston N, Currin A, Day PJ, Kell DB (2014) GeneGenie: optimised oligomer design for directed evolution. Nucleic Acids Res 12:W395–W400. doi:10.1093/nar/gku336

19. Knight CG, Platt M, Rowe W, Wedge DC, Khan F, Day P, McShea A, Knowles J, Kell DB (2009) Array-based evolution of DNA aptamers allows modelling of an explicit sequence-fitness landscape. Nucleic Acids Res 37(1):e6

20. Oates MJ, Corne DW, Kell DB (2003) The bimodal feature at large population sizes and high selection pressure: implications for directed evolution. In: Tan KC, Lim MH, Yao X, Wang L (eds) Recent advances in simulated evolution and learning. World Scientific, Singapore, pp 215–240

21. Fox RJ, Davis SC, Mundorff EC, Newman LM, Gavrilovic V, Ma SK, Chung LM, Ching C, Tam S, Muley S, Grate J, Gruber J, Whitman JC, Sheldon RA, Huisman GW (2007) Improving catalytic function by ProSAR-driven enzyme evolution. Nat Biotechnol 25(3):338–344

22. Nomenclature Committee of the International Union of Biochemistry (NC-IUB) (1985) Nomenclature for incompletely specified bases in nucleic acid sequences. Recommendations 1984. Eur J Biochem 150:1–5

Chapter 6

BASIC: A Simple and Accurate Modular DNA Assembly Method

Marko Storch, Arturo Casini, Ben Mackrow, Tom Ellis, and Geoff S. Baldwin

Abstract

Biopart Assembly Standard for Idempotent Cloning (**BASIC**) is a simple, accurate, and robust DNA assembly method. The method is based on linker-mediated DNA assembly and provides highly accurate DNA assembly with 99 % correct assemblies for four parts and 90 % correct assemblies for seven parts [1]. The BASIC standard defines a single entry vector for all parts flanked by the same prefix and suffix sequences and its idempotent nature means that the assembled construct is returned in the same format. Once a part has been adapted into the BASIC format it can be placed at any position within a BASIC assembly without the need for reformatting. This allows laboratories to grow comprehensive and universal part libraries and to share them efficiently. The modularity within the BASIC framework is further extended by the possibility of encoding ribosomal binding sites (RBS) and peptide linker sequences directly on the linkers used for assembly. This makes BASIC a highly versatile library construction method for combinatorial part assembly including the construction of promoter, RBS, gene variant, and protein-tag libraries. In comparison with other DNA assembly standards and methods, BASIC offers a simple robust protocol; it relies on a single entry vector, provides for easy hierarchical assembly, and is highly accurate for up to seven parts per assembly round [2].

Key words DNA assembly, Hierarchical, Idempotent, Combinatorial, Pathway engineering

1 Introduction

BASIC DNA assembly is based on linker-guided DNA assembly and includes an established standard which defines a design framework for linkers and a format for part storage. This BASIC standard requires the same integrated prefix (iP; 5′-TCTGGTGGGTCT CTGTCC-3′) and suffix (iS; 5′-GGCTCGGGAGACCTATCG-3′) sequences flanking each part (Fig. 1a). These sequences contain a *Bsa*I recognition site each, which are used to release parts from the storage vector resulting in different four base overhangs flanking the DNA part at both ends. These overhangs are used to

Randall A. Hughes (ed.), *Synthetic DNA: Methods and Protocols*, Methods in Molecular Biology, vol. 1472, DOI 10.1007/978-1-4939-6343-0_6, © Springer Science+Business Media New York 2017

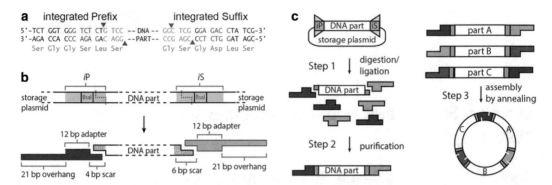

Fig. 1 BASIC standard and workflow. (**a**) Prefix (*iP*) and suffix (*iS*) sequences flanking each part including *Bsa*I cleavage sites (*red arrows*) for part release with specific four base overhangs. (**b**) Linker design and linker ligation mechanism. (**c**) BASIC workflow in three steps. Reprinted (adapted) with permission from [1]. Copyright 2015 American Chemical Society

ligate prefix- and suffix-specific linkers that are partially double stranded to facilitate ligation which subsequently provide long single-stranded and highly specific overhangs. The sequences of the overhangs then direct the accurate annealing of parts in a defined order within the assembly. The sequences of the linkers are derived from an online computational algorithm that ensures that they are orthogonal to the host genome sequence and do not contain secondary structures or proscribed restriction enzyme sequences [3, 4].

The BASIC assembly workflow contains three major steps (Fig. 1):

1. Linker ligation reaction (Subheading 3.3).

2. Part purification (Subheading 3.4).

3. DNA assembly step (Subheading 3.5).

The outlined BASIC workflow allows for a highly accurate DNA assembly, which can assemble four parts with 99 % and seven parts with 90 % accuracy [1].

Linkers required for the organization of the DNA assembly may also be used to encode functional elements of choice [1]. Three examples are described in Fig. 2:

1. Methylated linkers are used to reconstitute prefix and suffix sequences around a composition of parts during BASIC assembly. The resulting composition is thus returned as a single part in BASIC format flanked by *i*P and *i*S. The specific methylation of the *Bsa*I recognition sites prevents the cleavage of these linker sequences during the initial assembly round but is not maintained during replication of the first-stage DNA assembly in *E. coli*, rendering these prefix and suffix sites fully functional for a second round of DNA assembly.

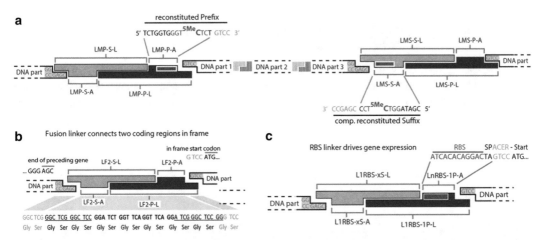

Fig. 2 BASIC functional linkers. (**a**) Methylated linkers LMP and LMS (Table 1) are used to reconstitute BASIC prefix and suffix sequences around compositions of parts. (**b**) Protein fusion linkers can be used to join protein domains to fusion proteins. (**c**) RBS encoded on linkers allows for simple RBS library creation via combinatorial linker design. Reprinted (adapted) with permission from [1]. Copyright 2015 American Chemical Society

2. Fusion linkers can be designed to encode for a peptide linker between two protein domains in frame to create a fusion protein between two BASIC parts. Fusion linker libraries encoding peptide linkers of varying length and flexibility allow for rapid protein engineering.

3. RBS linkers encode functional RBS sequences directly on the double-stranded portion of the linkers, driving translation of downstream open reading frame (ORF) parts. Linker libraries encoding RBS sequences of different strength are a powerful tool to tune gene expression within constructs assembled using BASIC.

Along with the standard protocol we provide detailing sections in italic for the construction of an example five-part plasmid containing the following parts in BASIC format (Genbank accession numbers provided in brackets): (A) Chloramphenicol resistance cassette (Cm) (KP223698); (B) Kanamycin resistance cassette (Kan) (KP223697); (C) MB1 origin (KP223695); (D) RFP expression cassette (KP223706); (E) GFP expression cassette (KP223703). These parts can also be obtained from Addgene (www.addgene.com). We use neutral linkers L2–L6 (materials section) to join these five parts (Fig. 3) (note that L6 is used instead of L1 to keep the linker sequences consistent with the original BASIC paper [1]).

To generate the assembled components (here red fluorescent protein (RFP) and green fluorescent protein (GFP)) as a reusable BASIC part they can be bracketed by the methylated linkers LMP and LMS (in place of L4 and L6, respectively; Table 1), which regenerate the prefix and suffix sequences.

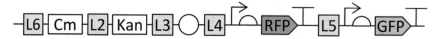

Fig. 3 Five-part test assembly RFP-GFP reporter plasmid. L2–L6 are used to assemble the five parts necessary to construct this fluorescent reporter plasmid from two resistance parts (chloramphenicol (Cm), kanamycin (Kan), one origin of replication part, and an RFP and GFP expression part). Reprinted (adapted) with permission from [1]. Copyright 2015 American Chemical Society

Table 1
Oligonucleotides for linkers

Name			Sequence 5′ → 3′
L2	L2S	L2S-L	*PO₄-CTCG*atcggtgtgtgaaaagtcagtatccagtcgtgtag
		L2S-A	*PO₄-*tttcacaccgat
	L2P	L2P-L	*PO₄-GGAC*aggtaataagaactacacgactggatactgact
		L2P-A	*PO₄-*ttcttattacct
L3	L3S	L3S-L	*PO₄-CTCG*atcacggcactacactcgttgctttatcggtat
		L3S-A	*PO₄-*tagtgccgtgat
	L3P	L3P-L	*PO₄-GGAC*tctgtaataacaataccgataaagcaacgagtg
		L3P-A	*PO₄-*tgttattacaga
L4	L4S	L4S-L	*PO₄-CTCG*acccacgactattgactgctctgagaaagttga
		L4S-A	*PO₄-*atagtcgtgggt
	L4P	L4P-L	*PO₄-GGAC*taatcgtaacaatcaactttctcagagcagtca
		L4P-A	*PO₄-*ttgttacgatta
L5	L5S	L5S-L	*PO₄-CTCG*agaagtagtgccacagacagtattgcttacgag
		L5S-A	*PO₄-*ggcactacttct
	L5P	L5P-L	*PO₄-GGAC*aggataaatcaactcgtaagcaatactgtctgt
		L5P-A	*PO₄-*ttgatttatcct
L6	L6S	L6S-L	*PO₄-CTCG*gtattgtaaagcacgaaacctacgataagagtg
		L6S-A	*PO₄-*gctttacaatac
	L6P	L6P-L	*PO₄-GGAC*aaggagaactgacactcttatcgtaggtttcgt
		L6P-A	*PO₄-*tcagttctcctt
LMP	LMP-S	LMP-S-L	*PO₄-CTCG*GGTAAGAACTCGCACTTCGTGGAAACACTATTA
		LMP-S-A	*PO₄-*CGAGTTCTTACC
	LMP-P	LMP-P-L	*PO₄-GGAC*AGAGACCCACCAGATAATAGTGTTTCCACGAAGTG
		LMP-P-A	*PO₄-*TCTGGTGGGT/iMe-dC/TCT
LMS	LMS-S	LMS-S-L	*PO₄-CTCG*GGAGACCTATCGGTAATAACAGTCCAATCTGGTGT
		LMS-S-A	*PO₄-*CGATAGGT/iMe-dC/TCC
	LMS-P	LMS-P-L	*PO₄-GGAC*GATTCCGAAGTTACACCAGATTGGACTGTTATTAC
		LMS-P-A	*PO₄-*AACTTCGGAATC

Oligonucleotides constituting neutral BASIC linkers (L2–6) and methylated linkers (LMP, LMS). BsaI cut site annealing regions are shown in bold; linker annealing regions are shown in italic. Oligonucleotides are ordered 5′ phosphorylated, HPLC purified and with an internal 5′-C methylation for LMP-P-A and LMS-S-A

2   Materials

1. Oligonucleotide buffer: 10 mM Tris–HCl pH 7.9 (25 °C), dH$_2$O.

2. Linker annealing buffer: 10 mM Tris–HCl pH 7.9 (25 °C), 100 mM NaCl, 10 mM MgCl$_2$, dH$_2$O.

3. 10× NEB4 buffer: 500 mM KCH$_3$COO, 200 mM Tris-CH$_3$COO, 100 mM Mg(CH$_3$COO)$_2$, 10 mM DTT, pH 7.9 (25 °C), dH$_2$O.

4. 10× BSA: 10 mg/ml BSA (NEB).

5. 10× ATP: 10 mM ATP in Tris–HCl, pH 7.9 (25 °C).

6. *Bsa*I: *Bsa*I-HF (NEB), 20 units/μl.

7. T4 ligase: T4 DNA ligase (NEB), 400 units/μl.

8. dH$_2$O.

9. 70 % Ethanol.

10. Magnetic beads: Agencourt AMPure XP (Beckman Coulter).

11. Magnetic plate, 96 well (AM10050 Ambion, Applied Biosystems).

12. 96-Well Falcon plate, U-shaped bottom.

13. Phusion Polymerase kit (NEB).

14. PJet 1.2 CloneJet PCR cloning kit (Life Technologies).

15. LB medium: 10 g/l Tryptone, 5 g/l yeast extract, 10 g/l NaCl, dH$_2$O.

16. LB agar: 10 g/l Tryptone, 5 g/l yeast extract, 10 g/l NaCl, 15 g/l agar, dH$_2$O.

17. SOC medium: 20 g/l Tryptone, 5 g/l yeast extract, 0.36 g/l glucose, 0.58 g/l NaCl, 0.19 g/l KCl, 2 g/l MgCl$_2$·6H$_2$O, 2.46 g/l MgSO$_4$·7H$_2$O, dH$_2$O.

18. Chemically competent DH5α strain (Life Technologies/in-house prepared [5]).

3   Methods

Methods are subdivided into sections addressing BASIC part preparation (Subheading 3.1), linker preparation (Subheading 3.2), linker ligation reaction (Subheading 3.3), part purification (Subheading 3.4), DNA assembly step (Subheading 3.5), heat-shock transformation into *E. coli* (Subheading 3.6), and conclusion on screening for correct colonies (Subheading 3.7).

3.1   BASIC Part Preparation

1. Adding prefix and suffix sequences to each part by PCR: Add the prefix sense sequence (iP; 5′-TCTGGTGGGTCTC TGTCC-3′) to the 5′ end of the part-specific forward primer

and the reverse complement of the suffix sequence (iS; 5′-CGATAGGTCTCCCGAGCC-3′) to the 5′ end of the part-specific reverse primer. Clone the PCR product into pJet 1.2 according to the manufacturer's protocol, which provides a quick and low-background cloning procedure (*see* **Note 1**).

2. Sequence-verify each part in its storage vector. Depending on the part size the pJet 1.2-specific primers (pJET1.2 forward: 5′-CGACTCACTATAGGGAGAGCGGC-3′; pJET1.2 reverse: 5′-AAGAACATCGATTTTCCATGGCAG-3′; supplied with the CloneJet kit) can provide sufficient sequence coverage. Importantly, ensure that both prefix and suffix sites are completely sequence verified. Since no PCR is used throughout the BASIC assembly process, there is less of an imperative to sequence the final construct.

Sequence files of parts A–E can be accessed online via their Genbank entry numbers and ordered through Addgene (www.addgene.com).

3.2 Linker Preparation

1. Choose linkers you like to use for your assembly from the original BASIC paper [1], or use R2o DNA Design software (http://www.r2odna.com/) [4], to create your own orthogonal linker sets (*see* **Note 2**). For each linker order the corresponding four 5′ phosphorylated oligonucleotides, HPLC purified from your preferred oligonucleotide supplier (*see* **Note 3**). *For the five-part assembly use the five neutral linkers L2–L6 consisting of four oligonucleotides each as described in Table 1 (materials).*

2. Prepare 100 μM stock solutions of all linker oligonucleotides in oligonucleotide buffer.

3. Mix pairwise oligonucleotides that make up the respective prefix (e.g., L2P = L2P-L + L2P-A) and the suffix (e.g., L2S = L2S-L + L2S-A) modules of the linkers in linker annealing buffer to 1 μM in 1.5 ml Eppendorf tubes (e.g., add 2 μl of each oligonucleotide stock solution (100 μM) to 196 μl of linker annealing buffer and mix). Heat the linker solution to 95 °C in a heating block and allow slow cooling to room temperature after switching off the heating block (alternatively use slow ramp down on PCR cycler). These ready-to-use linker solutions can be stored for 4 weeks at 4 °C or –20 °C.

For the five-part assembly prepare L2P = L2P-L + L2P-A; L2S = L2S-L + L2S-A; L3P = L3P-L + L3P-A; … L6S = L6S-L + L6S-A.

3.3 Linker Ligation Reaction

1. For each part mix a separate linker ligation reaction in a 200 μl PCR tube: 5 μl H_2O, 3 μl 10× NEB4 buffer, 3 μl 10× BSA (10 mg/ml), 3 μl 10× ATP (10 mM), 5 μl of prefix linker mix, 5 μl of suffix linker mix, ~ 75fmol of part DNA (usually 1 μl), top up with H_2O to 28.5 μl. Add 1 μl of *Bsa*I-HF (20 units),

add 0.5 μl of T4 ligase (200 units), mix by pipetting up and down, and incubate in PCR machine running the linker ligation program: 37 °C for 60 min, 20 °C for 20 min, and 65 °C for 25 min; store at 4 °C (*see* **Notes 4** and **5**).

For the five-part assembly test, each part is mixed with corresponding prefix and suffix linkers in five individual part-specific linker ligation reactions, according to assembly plan in Fig. 3, e.g., linker reaction mix including 1 μl of part A (Cm, normalized to 200 ng/μl) + 5 μl of L6P + 5 μl L2S; 1 μl of part B (Kan, normalized to 200 ng/μl) + 5 μl of L2P + 5 μl L3S; ... 1 μl of part E (GFP, normalized to 200 ng/μl) + 5 μl of L5P + 5 μl L6S.

Remember*—Prefix or suffix linker nomenclature refers to whether the linker will be added onto the prefix or suffix overhang of a digested part.

3.4 Part Purification Step

The linker annealing reactions will be purified from remaining free oligonucleotides and reaction mix. Each purification will take place in one well of a Falcon 96-well U-shaped bottom plate, using 54 μl Agencourt Ampure XP magnetic beads (or similar) on an Ambion 96-well magnetic stand (*see* **Note 6**).

Steps are described for one part and will in practice be done in parallel for the number of parts relevant to the particular assembly project. *In our example of a five-part assembly, five purification reactions are performed in parallel.*

1. For each linker ligation reaction, add 54 μl of resuspended magnetic bead solution into a well, add the 30 μl linker ligation reaction, and mix by pipetting up and down ten times. Wait for 5 min to allow DNA binding to magnetic beads.

2. Place 96-well plate onto magnet and wait for 2 min for stable magnetic bead rings forming at the well bottom. Be careful not to disturb these rings in the next steps.

3. Remove liquid (~85 μl) and discard.

4. First wash step: Add 190 μl 70% ethanol.

5. First wash step: Remove liquid (~200 μl) and discard.

6. Second wash step: Add 190 μl 70% ethanol.

7. Second wash step: Remove liquid (~200 μl) and discard.

8. Let wells dry for 5–10 min (without lid).

9. Place 96-well plate off the magnet and add 40 μl of H₂O. Mix ten times. Wait for 1 min.

10. Place 96-well plate back onto magnet and wait for 2 min for magnetic bead rings to form at the well bottom.

11. Purified DNA is released into H₂O and can be transferred into a labeled fresh Eppendorf tube each (transfer 30 μl, leaving ~10 μl behind). Avoid disrupting the ring and do not take up any of the magnetic beads.

3.5 DNA Assembly Step

Combine 1 μl of each part in total volume of 10 μl with 1× NEB 4 buffer and 1× BSA in 200 μl PCR tube (*see* **Notes 7** and **8**).

Add 1 μl 10× NEB4 and 1 μl 10× BSA (10 mg/ml) to a 200 μl PCR tube.

1. Add (8–*x*) μl H$_2$O (*x*=number of parts in assembly).

2. Add 1 μl of each purified part and mix ten times.

3. Incubate 10 μl reaction in PCR cycler: 50 °C for 60 min; store at 4 °C.

For the five-part assembly, 1 μl of each purified, linker-ligated part is added to 3 μl of H$_2$O, 1 μl of 10× NEB4, and 1 μl of 10× BSA.

3.6 Transformation of Assembled DNA

Using highly competent cells (>10^9 CFU/μg pUC19) is crucial for returning many colonies for assemblies of more than five parts (*see* **Note 9**).

1. Transfer 5 μl assembly mix into 1.5 ml microfuge tube and chill on ice.

2. Thaw chemically competent cells on ice.

3. Transfer 45 μl of competent cells into chilled 1.5 ml microfuge tube with 5 μl of assembly mix.

4. Incubate on ice for 20 min, heat-shock in 42 °C water bath for 45 s, and chill on ice again for 2 min.

5. Add 600 μl pre-warmed SOC medium to 1.5 ml microfuge tube and incubate shaking at 600 rpm at 37° for at least 60 min.

6. Pre-warm LB-agar plate with appropriate selection antibiotics.

7. Spin down cells at 10,000×*g* for 1 min, and discard 500 μl media supernatant.

8. Resuspend cells in the remaining ~150 μl medium and spread onto pre-warmed LB-agar plate.

9. Incubate overnight at 37 °C.

For the five-part assembly use LB-agar plates with 50 μg/ml kanamycin and 50 μg/ml chloramphenicol. One would expect more than 500 colonies, so it is advisable to split the cells after step 7 *into 10 and 90 % and plate both volumes on individual LB-agar plates.*

3.7 Screening for Correct Assemblies

Given the high accuracy of BASIC assembly usually just a few colonies have to be screened via colony PCR. Conveniently standard linkers used to connect the assembly parts can serve as standard priming sites. Combinations of such linker-directed forward and reverse primers will produce PCR products that reflect the cumulative size of the parts in between a given forward and reverse primer pair. Plasmids from correctly identified colonies may also be sequence verified (*see* **Notes 10** and **11**).

Table 2
Oligonucleotides for construct validation via colony PCR

Oligonucleotide name	Sequence 5′ → 3′
V-L6-F	GCACGAAACCTACGATAAGAGTGTCAG
V-L2-R	GAACTACACGACTGGATACTGACTTTTCACAC
V-L3-R	CAATACCGATAAAGCAACGAGTGTAGTGC
V-L4-R	CAATCAACTTTCTCAGAGCAGTCAATAGTCG
V-L5-R	CAACTCGTAAGCAATACTGTCTGTGGC

Ordered as standard primers (desalted)

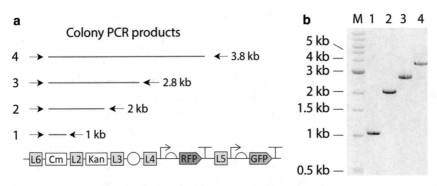

Fig. 4 Colony PCR screen for correct five-part assembly. (**a**) Primer pairs from Table 2 binding to linker sequences will result in specific bands, when the construct is assembled correctly as shown for five-part assembly in (**b**). Reprinted (adapted) with permission from [1]. Copyright 2015 American Chemical Society

For example, the five-part assembly colony PCR is performed using a forward primer annealing to linker L6 (V-L6-F) and reverse primers annealing to linker L2, L3, L4, L5 (V-L2-R, V-L3-R, V-L4-R, V-L5-R) (Table 2, Fig. 4). Single colonies are dissolved in 10 μl H$_2$O and 2 μl are used in PCR reactions. Primers are designed for a T$_m$ = 65 °C and Phusion or Pfu DNA Polymerases may be used in these standard PCR reactions. The PCR program suggested for the five-part example with Phusion DNA Polymerase consists of the following steps: 3 min at 98 °C, 30 cycles of 10 s at 98 °C, 30 s at 65 °C, 2.5 min at 72 °C, and a final elongation step of 10 min at 72 °C. Running these reactions on a 1 % agarose gel will show a banding pattern reflecting the size and order of parts in the correct assembly (Fig. 4b). In case of the five-part RFP-GFP reporter construct the positive colonies may also be identified by measuring the fluorescence profile of the colonies with methods accessible to the user (GFP signal measured on blue box for DNA gels; GFP and RFP signals measured on fluorescence plate reader; RFP expression will render colonies red, visible by eye after 2 days of colony growth).

4   Notes

1. BASIC part preparation: Since *Bsa*I digestion is used to release each part from its storage vector and expose linker attachment sites (four base overhangs), parts must not contain *Bsa*I sites. *Bsa*I sites are rare, but in case a part of interest contains such a site standard mutagenesis methods can be applied to introduce a silent mutation that removes the *Bsa*I recognition site. Standard PCR methods are used to attach prefix and suffix sequences to new parts before cloning them into pJet1.2 vector (CloneJet, Life Technologies). Alternatively directly synthesized double-stranded DNA (e.g., gBlocks from IDT), which provides an economical solution for part sizes up to 2 kbp, can be ordered including prefix and suffix sequences (Fig. 1) excluding any internal *Bsa*I sites and then cloned into the pJet 1.2 vector according to supplier's protocol. In cases where origins of replication are included within a part, storage in pJet 1.2 may result in unstable plasmids. In these cases the flanking prefix and suffix sequences are generated via PCR. If the part also contains a selection marker the resulting PCR product is blunt ligated. If the origin part does not contain a selection cassette the PCR product may be joined with a selection cassette via Gibson Assembly. In principle any other storage backbone could be chosen to house the DNA part, as long as it allows for part release with the specific overhangs (Fig. 1), and does not result in any other digestion products that show the prefix- or suffix-specific four base overhangs after *Bsa*I digestion. Besides the high efficiency in cloning parts into pJet 1.2, this vector also contains an AmpR cassette that is cleaved at an internal *Bsa*I restriction site, which will reduce the background from surviving BASIC selection cassettes in storage vector. A further strategy to address background issues is to generate PCR products with primers inclusive of the prefix and suffix sequences, thus incorporating them into the part. Subsequent addition of parts as such PCR products into the linker ligation step avoids any carry through of background plasmids during the final BASIC assembly. Usually the benefit of sequence-verified parts in storage vector with standardized concentrations saves on time and out-weights this minor improvement with *ad hoc*-prepared BASIC-compatible PCR products.

2. Linkers (methylated/RBS/fusion linkers): The design of linkers that perform well in BASIC's assembly step is fundamental for high accuracy and efficiency of the assembly process. Foundation for their design principles was laid through our work on the MODAL and BASIC methods and our freely available online linker design tool R2o DNA Designer ([3, 4], http://www.r2odna.com/). In brief, linker sequences are

optimized to contain no unwanted motifs or complementarity and perform well during the linker annealing and the final assembly step. A complete list of linker sequences along with the oligonucleotides needed to build them is provided in the supplementary material of our BASIC paper [1]. New orthogonal linker sets can be created straightforwardly with the R2o DNA Design software tool [4]. Special linkers containing functional sequences like RBS and peptide fusion linkers are designed manually and checked for being orthogonal to other linkers being used within the same assemblies, via the R2O DNA Design reverse mode.

3. Linker oligonucleotide phosphorylation: Alternatively to ordering 5′ phosphorylated linker oligonucleotides, one can include T4-polynucleotide kinase in the assembly reaction, which will provide some level of phosphorylation allowing the connection of linkers to the part during the linker ligation reaction. While the up-front cost for buying HPLC-purified and phosphorylated linker oligonucleotides is relatively high, they will last for thousands of BASIC reactions and their contribution to per reaction cost is negligible (main cost factors being enzymes). For the purposes of evaluating BASIC it is possible to order standard primer oligonucleotides and include T4 PNK, but there may be some loss of overall efficiency. Methylation of the adapter oligonucleotides for the iP and iS linkers is also added during synthesis at negligible cost, but requires a slightly larger synthesis scale than for primer oligonucleotides.

4. Normalized part concentration: Newly domesticated BASIC parts are sequence verified and adjusted to concentrations so that 1 μl would provide a final 2.5 nM concentration in the linker annealing reaction. The required concentration is approximated to ~50 ng/μl per 1 kbp of complete plasmid size. For instance for a GFP part of around 1 kbp stored in a pJet 1.2 backbone of around 3 kbp, the plasmid solution would be normalized to ~200 ng/μl to ease workflow and automation.

5. Enzyme activity: A complete digest of storage vector is central to a highly efficient and accurate BASIC assembly, since undigested selection cassettes in storage plasmids can give rise to background in single selection scenarios. When setting up BASIC assembly for the first time or when using fresh batches of *Bsa*I-HF and T4 ligase we recommend running 5 μl of finished linker ligation reaction (after Subheading 3.3) or purified parts (after Subheading 3.4) on a 1 % agarose gel to check for complete digest of the storage plasmid. When storage vector digest is incomplete, extending the digestion temperature step during the linker ligation PCR cycle protocol (end of Subheading 3.3) usually provides a more complete digest

(ranges from 37 °C for 1 h up to 4 h). Furthermore, the ratio between *Bsa*I restriction enzyme and T4 ligase can be re-adjusted by reducing the amount of T4 ligase (optional dilution in diluent A from NEB).

6. Part purification: We found that spin columns did not provide sufficient removal of un-ligated oligonucleotides, which severely compromises the overall assembly efficiency. Therefore the protocol requires using the AMPure purification mag bead system and we also recommend using the Falcon U-shaped 96-well plates, since we found that other plates did not allow as stable magnetic bead rings to form while on the Ambion magnet stand. This is important for high yields of DNA from the purification step. Single-tube magnetic stands might work as well, but we did not test their efficiency. If one wants to control for the return of DNA from this purification step, running the purified samples on a 1 % agarose gel will show both the presence of purified DNA parts and the efficiency of the linker annealing on storage plasmid released parts (part corresponding DNA band vs. complete storage vector band; note that pJet 1.2 storage vector (3 kbp) will be digested at the AMP gene further into a 1.3 and 1.7 kbp fragment).

7. Buffer system: We used NEB4 buffer and BSA for historical reasons. Currently available buffer systems like NEB CutSmart (includes BSA) should work just as well.

8. DNA amount in assembly step: Depending on the number of parts, one can increase the amount of DNA parts going into the final assembly to maximize the number of colonies returned after transformation. For instance in a five-part assembly 1.6 μl of each purified part can be used and will increase the number of returned colonies. While maximizing the number of colonies is not so important for simple 2–7-part assemblies, it becomes crucial when construct diversity shall be covered after plating combinatorial assemblies where individual clones will differ in promoter, RBS, or gene variants within the same assembly framework.

9. Chemically competent DH5α cells: Using BASIC successfully for up to seven parts requires highly competent cells of 10^9 CFU/μg pUC19. Such highly competent cells can be ordered from different vendors or prepared in-house. We are using the Inoue protocol [5] to prepare high-efficiency chemically competent *E. coli DH5α* cells. We adapted the original protocol by using 300 ml SOC medium for the final outgrowth to OD600 0.3–0.55 at 18 °C, shaking at 220 rpm.

10. Standard test primers: Since standard linker sequences are used to assemble parts in BASIC format they efficiently serve as watermarks for test PCR primers to confer the presence

and order of parts. Depending on the construct design we routinely choose primers from a linker-specific primer list [1] to confirm positive clones via colony PCR. Since all parts are usually sequence verified in their storage plasmids and no PCR amplification step is used throughout the BASIC workflow, it is highly unlikely that the part sequences would carry mutations in the assembled construct. The complete standardization of the workflow including standard test colony PCR primers leverages the advantages of BASIC assembly especially for high-throughput library construction.

11. Single vs. double selection: We found undigested resistance cassettes for selection still in their storage vector to be the main source of background colonies after transformation, while incorrect assemblies are extremely rare events. Since even very small amounts of undigested resistance cassettes will contribute a background level of around 40 colonies for any assembly we devised double selection as a standard strategy in our lab. While for less than five-part assemblies the ~40 background colonies do not reduce accuracy within thousands of correct colonies, especially for seven-part assemblies when overall colonies returned from transformation are below 100, this source of background forces one to screen more colonies in order to identify the correct ones. When two independent selection marker parts (e.g., KanR and CmR) are included in the overall assembly strategy, then double selection (on KanR and CmR) lifts overall accuracy up to 90% for seven-part assemblies—providing BASIC with a very high accuracy when compared to other techniques.

References

1. Storch M, Casini A, Mackrow B et al (2015) BASIC: a new biopart assembly standard for idempotent cloning provides accurate, single-tier DNA assembly for synthetic biology. ACS Synth Biol 4(7):781–787. doi:10.1021/sb500356

2. Casini A, Storch M, Baldwin G, Ellis T (2015) Bricks and blueprints: methods and standards for DNA assembly. Nat Rev Mol Cell Biol 16:568–576. doi:10.1038/nrm4014

3. Casini A, Macdonald JT, Jonghe JD et al (2013) One-pot DNA construction for synthetic biology: the Modular Overlap-Directed Assembly with Linkers (MODAL) strategy. Nucleic Acids Res 42:e7. doi:10.1093/nar/gkt915

4. Casini A, Christodoulou G, Freemont P et al (2014) R2oDNA designer: computational design of biologically neutral synthetic DNA sequences. ACS Synth Biol 3:525–528. doi:10.1021/sb4001323

5. Inoue H, Nojima H, Okayama H (1990) High efficiency transformation of Escherichia coli with plasmids. Gene 96:23–28. doi:10.1016/0378-1119(90)90336-P

Chapter 7

Enzymatic Synthesis of Single-Stranded Clonal Pure Oligonucleotides

Cosimo Ducani and Björn Högberg

Abstract

Single-stranded oligonucleotides, or oligodeoxyribonucleotides (ODNs), are very important in several fields of science such as molecular biology, diagnostics, nanotechnology, and gene therapy. They are usually chemically synthesized. Here we describe an enzymatic method which enables us to synthesize pure oligonucleotides which can be up to several hundred long bases.

Key words Enzymatic DNA synthesis, RCA, MOSIC, Single-stranded oligonucleotides, DNA nanotechnology

1 Introduction

ODNs are typically synthesized using solid phase, phosphoramidite polymer chemistries [1]. These synthetic technologies, although impressive, cannot compete with the capacity of natural polymerases in terms of producing pure, long, and accurate DNA polymers at high synthesis scales [2]. Moreover, it has been shown that synthetic DNA products contain a high percentage of impurities including oligonucleotides with internal deletions or insertions, not completely deprotected or partially modified ODNs, and the number of synthetic errors observed typically increases with the length of the synthetic products [3]. High-performance liquid chromatography (HPLC) or polyacrylamide gel electrophoresis (PAGE) based purification methods increases the cost of ODNs production but ensures merely an enrichment of the desired products [4, 5]. To overcome these limitations enzymatic methods for ODNs production have been developed. For instance both polymerase chain reaction (PCR) [6, 7] and rolling circle amplification (RCA) technologies [8] have been adopted for producing DNA oligomers but in both cases the production relies on the use of synthetic oligonucleotide primers which can introduce errors

Randall A. Hughes (ed.), *Synthetic DNA: Methods and Protocols*, Methods in Molecular Biology, vol. 1472,
DOI 10.1007/978-1-4939-6343-0_7, © Springer Science+Business Media New York 2017

which are then propagated in the final product. In addition, PCR provides double-stranded DNA, which means that extra steps must be taken to remove the unwanted complementary strand.

Here we describe a detailed protocol to perform the "monoclonal stoichiometric" (MOSIC) method [9], which is based on the use of bacteria and/or enzymatic reactions to produce very pure oligonucleotides in a certain stoichiometry and when required, also several hundred bases long.

The main idea underlying this technology is to use a clonal, long, single-stranded DNA template (called pseudogene) to assemble the desired oligo sequences with small hairpin structures in between them. The pseudogene can be ordered from gene-synthesis services or assembled in house in its double-stranded form. Through sequencing and error correction it is possible to obtain 100 % pure clones with exactly the desired sequence. We have developed two different strategies to amplify the pseudogene in single-stranded form: one based on RCA and the other one on helper phage DNA rescue. In both approaches we treat the amplicons with a Type-IIs restriction enzyme (BseGI in our case) that specifically digests the hairpin, releasing the desired single-stranded oligonucleotides from the template, clonally pure, in a required stoichiometry and in large scale.

2 Materials

2.1 Equipment

1. Bacterial cultivation equipment (shakers, autoclave, incubators).
2. Centrifuges both benchtop and floor models.
3. Freeze dryer.
4. Speed vacuum system.
5. Thermocycler.
6. Agarose and polyacrylamide gel electrophoresis equipment.
7. UV transilluminator and UV gel imager.

2.2 RCA Strategy

1. Phagemid DNA containing the MOSIC pseudogene.
2. Enzymes: BsaI-HF restriction enzyme or another non-palindromic restriction enzyme, nicking endonucleases Nb.BsrDI and Nt.BspQI, T4 DNA ligase, phi29 DNA polymerase, T4 gene 32 single-stranded binding protein, BseGI restriction enzyme.
3. Elution buffer: 5 mM Tris–HCl (pH 8) or deionized water.
4. 10× CutSmart buffer (NEB): 500 mM potassium acetate, 200 mM Tris-acetate, 100 mM magnesium acetate, 10 mg/ml BSA (pH 7.9).

5. 10× Tango buffer: 330 mM Tris-acetate (pH 7.9 at 37 °C), 100 mM magnesium acetate, 660 mM potassium acetate, 1 mg/ml BSA.

6. Gel extraction kit.

7. Strata-clean resin (Agilent).

8. Sep-Pak C18 cartridges (Waters).

2.3 Helper Phage Strategy

1. LB medium: dissolve 10 g tryptone, 5 g yeast extract, and 10 g NaCl in 950 ml deionized water, adjust the pH of the medium to 7.0 using 1 N NaOH and bring volume up to 1 l, autoclave on liquid cycle for 20 min at 15 psi. Allow solution to cool to 55 °C, and add antibiotic when required.

2. LB agar: prepare LB medium as above, but add 15 g/l agar before autoclaving.

3. Antibiotics: ampicillin and kanamycin.

4. 2× YT medium: 16.0 g/l tryptone, 10.0 g/l yeast extract, 5.0 g/l NaCl, adjusted to pH 7.0 with NaOH.

5. Phagemid vector with pseudogene insert.

6. Helper phage VCM13.

7. 1 M $MgCl_2$ sterile.

8. PEG 8000.

9. 10 mM Tris–HCl (pH 8).

10. Phage Prep Buffer 2 (PPB2): 0.2 M NaOH and 1% SDS.

11. Phage Prep Buffer 3 (PPB3): 3 M KOAc pH 5.5 titrated with glacial acetic acid.

12. BseGI restriction enzyme.

13. 5× T4 DNA Ligase Buffer: 250 mM Tris–HCl (pH 7.6), 50 mM $MgCl_2$, 5 mM ATP, 5 mM DTT, 25% (w/v) polyethylene glycol-8000.

14. 10× NEBuffer 3.1: 1 M NaCl, 500 mM Tris–HCl, 100 mM $MgCl_2$, 1 μg/ml BSA (pH 7.9).

15. 70% ethanol.

16. 100% ethanol.

17. Electrophoresis: quality control through PAGE or agarose gel:

    (a) 20× TBE buffer (pH 8.13–8.23): in 100 ml of deionized water dissolve 54 g of Tris(hydroxymethyl)aminomethane, 27.5 g of boric acid, and 2.92 g ethylenediaminetetraacetic acid (EDTA), then add deionized water up to 250 ml.

    (b) Orange Dye Solution: orange G 0.02% (w/v), 10% glycerol, 90% formamide.

    (c) 10,000× SYBR Gold.

(d) 100 bp or 10 bp ladder (GeneRuler Ultra Low Range or similar).

(e) 10–20% denaturing PAGE (20% formamide, 8 M urea): for 15 ml of gel solution dissolve 7.2 g urea into 3.75 or 7.5 ml 40% acrylamide–Bis Solution, 19:1 (Bio-Rad) (for 10 or 20% PAGE respectively) and 0.75 ml of 20× TBE (warming at 60 °C and stirring the solution will help all the components to dissolve completely). Leave the solution cooling down and add 3 ml of 100% formamide. Add deionized water up to 15 ml. For the gel polymerization add 70 μl of 10% ammonium persulfate and 7 μl TEMED (N,N,N',N'-Tetramethylethylenediamine).

(f) AGAROSE GEL: 2% agarose, 10 mM $MgCl_2$, 1 μg/ml ethidium bromide, 0.5× TBE buffer.

3   Methods

3.1   In Silico Pseudogene Design and E. coli Colony Preparation

1. Design the desired oligonucleotide sequences followed by the 23-base hairpin sequence, CATCCGTGGGAACCAC GGATGNN, where NN have to be complementary to the last two bases of the sequence preceding the hairpin. The hairpin contains the restriction sequence (GGATG) for the restriction enzyme BseGI (Fig. 1).

2. Insert, upstream of the initial hairpin sequence, the restriction site for pseudogene linearization (BsaI-HF, GGTCTC) and the nicking site for nicking endonuclease Nb.BsrDI (GCAATG), while downstream the last hairpin another sequence for BsaI-HF (this time inverted: GAGACC) and a nicking endonuclease sequence for Nt.BspQI (GCTCTTC) (see Note 1).

3. Order the pseudogene from a gene synthesis company which will be provided in double-stranded form inserted in a plasmid DNA vector (see Note 2).

4. Transform JM109 *E. coli* cells with the phagemid DNA. The transformation can be performed using standard electroporation or heat shock protocols. Several dilutions (from 1:10 to 1:100) of transformed cells are plated on a LB agar petri dish containing the antibiotic specific for the vector resistance. 5 ml LB liquid cultures containing the same antibiotic are inoculated with single colonies. 4 ml of the colony is used for miniprep protocol to extract the plasmid of cell culture, while the 1 ml is stored in the fridge for an eventual glycerol stock solution.

5. Colonies are screened by digesting the extract plasmid DNA with BsaI-HF restriction enzyme (or the chosen palindromic restriction enzyme). Digestion products are run on 1% agarose gel. Only colonies positive for the insert corresponding to the pseudogene will be used for glycerol stock and can be stored at –80 °C.

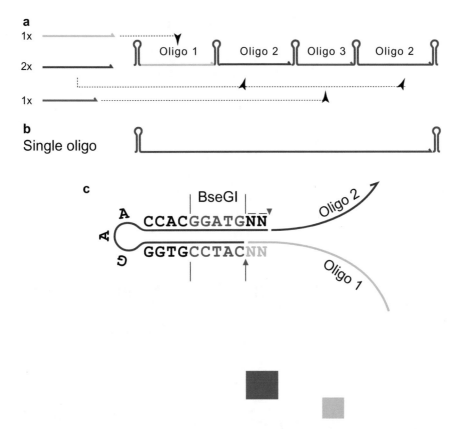

Fig. 1 Schematic representation of a pseudogene construction. (**a**) Assembling of short oligonucleotides in a certain stoichiometry. (**b**) Pseudogene made by a single long oligonucleotide. Restriction and nicking site are placed upstream of the first hairpin and downstream the last one. (**c**) Structure and sequence of the inter-oligonucleotide hairpin

6. Streak on a LB agar petri dish glycerol stock of *E. coli* cells previously transformed and screened for the pseudogene to get single colonies and incubate the petri dish overnight at 37 °C. The day after the synthesis of MOSIC oligonucleotides can be performed. This can be done in two different strategies: by RCA or by using a helper phage protocol.

3.2 RCA Strategy

1. Pick a single colony by using a sterile pipette tip and inoculate in a 15 ml falcon tube a 5 ml LB agar containing the appropriate antibiotic. Incubate overnight the culture at 37 °C shaking at 200 rpm.

2. Perform a standard miniprep protocol to extract the plasmid DNA. Elute in a final volume of 30 µl of elution buffer or deionized water. Measure the concentration of phagemid DNA by NanoDrop or plate reader and check its quality by running a 1.5 % agarose gel.

3. Pseudogene linearization: Digest the plasmid DNA by using BsaI-HF (or the chosen restriction enzyme for linearization) using a concentration of 20–50 ng/μl of plasmid DNA and 0.25 U/μl of BsaI-HF. In a typical linearization experiment 0.5–1 ml total volume reaction is used in 1× CutSmart buffer (NEB) (*see* **Note 3**). Load the digestion products in a 1.5 % agarose gel (EtBr 1 μg/ml) and run 120 V for 1:30 h (Fig. 2a). Using a UV transilluminator, excise the band corresponding to the expected length of the pseudogene from the gel and use a gel extraction kit to extract the linear pseudogene from the gel. Elute in 30 μl of elution buffer.

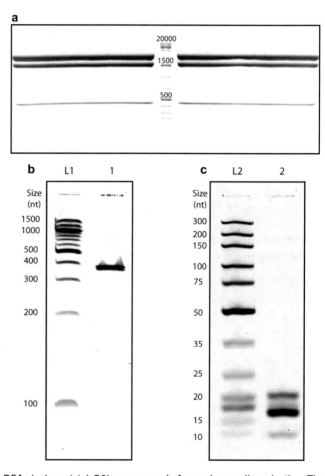

Fig. 2 RCA strategy. (**a**) 1.5 % agarose gel of pseudogene linearization. The faster band has to be excised and the DNA gel extracted. (**b**) Denaturing 10 % polyacrylamide gel of MOSIC oligonucleotide 378-base long provided by BseGI digestion of RCA products (*1*), 100 bp DNA ladder (*L1*); (**c**) Denaturing 20 % polyacrylamide gel of MOSIC oligonucleotides 21 and 14 bases long with the more intense band in between corresponding to the cutter hairpins (*2*), 10 bp DNA ladder (*L2*)

4. Pseudogene circularization: Ligate linear pseudogene (5 ng/μl) in 1× T4 DNA Ligase Buffer and T4 ligase 0.5 U/μl. A typical circularization volume is 20 μl. Incubate the reaction mixture at 22 °C for 30–60 min. Perform heat inactivation of the ligase at 65 °C for 20 min.

5. Pseudogene nicking: Dilute the ligation mixture five volumes (final pseudogene concentration 1 ng/μl) in 1× NEBuffer 3.1. Add 0.5 U/μl nicking endonuclease Nt.BspQI and incubate for 90 min at 50 °C. Following this incubation add 0.5 U/μl nicking endonuclease Nb.BsrDI and incubate for 90 min at 65 °C (*see* **Notes 4** and **5**). Heat-inactivate the enzymes by incubating the reaction mixture at 80 °C for 20 min.

6. Rolling Circle Replication: Prepare the rolling circle amplification by mixing, in a PCR tube, 0.1–0.25 ng/μl nicked circular pseudogene, 1× phi29 DNA polymerase buffer, 1 mM dNTP mix, 0.1–0.25 μg/μl T4 gene 32 single-stranded DNA binding protein, and 0.5 U/μl phi29 DNA polymerase (the reaction can be performed in 1.5 ml tubes in case of higher scale DNA oligonucleotide production). Incubate the reaction overnight at 30 °C. Phi29 DNA polymerase will amplify the pseudogene in single-stranded form as repeated concatemers [10] (*see* **Notes 6** and **7**).

7. Hairpin digestion: Digest the RCA product in a PCR tube by diluting it (2–4 μl in 10 μl reaction) in 1× Tango buffer and adding 1 U/μl BseGI restriction enzyme. Incubate the reaction mixture at 55 °C overnight (*see* **Note 8**). In case of high scale DNA oligo production the reaction can be performed in a 1.5 ml Eppendorf tube.

8. Quality control: Digestion products are first mixed with orange dye solution (1–5 μl of digestion products with orange dye solution up to 10–20 μl) and heat at 75 °C for 15 min, then loaded when still warm on a denaturing polyacrylamide gel (10% for oligonucleotides longer than 100 bases and 20% for oligonucleotides between 10 and 100 base long). The electrophoresis is performed with 1× TBE as running buffer (also warmed at 50 °C before being poured in the gel tank) at 150 or 180 V (for 10% and 20% PAGE respectively) until the orange dye is at the bottom of the gel. The gel is stained in 1× SYBR Gold for 10 min on a rocking shaker and visualized, afterwards, by UV camera (Fig. 2b, c).

9. Protein Removal: (Optional Step) Remove enzymes from the RCA digest reaction by running it through StrataClean Resin following the manufacturer's instructions.

10. Desalting step: Desalt oligonucleotides from the RCA digest by Sep-Pak C18 cartridges following the manufacturer's instructions. Lyophilize them overnight by using freeze dryer

first, then resuspend in 1 ml milliQ water (taking care to wash the walls of the falcon tubes thoroughly) and transfer the solution to an Eppendorf tube and lyophilize again by speed-vacuum concentrator (this will reduce loss of DNA after the first lyophilization).

3.3 Helper Phage Strategy

1. Pick a single colony by using a sterile pipette tip and inoculate in a 250 ml flask a 25 ml LB containing the appropriate antibiotic. Incubate overnight the culture at 37 °C shaking at 200 rpm.

2. With 3 ml of the saturated overnight culture inoculate four 2 l flasks containing 300-ml cultures of 2× YT medium containing the appropriate antibiotic, and add 1.5 ml of sterile 1 M $MgCl_2$.

3. Incubate the culture at 37 °C with shaking at 250 rpm and monitor the OD_{600} during the cell growth. Add VCSM13 helper phage at $OD_{600} = 0.45$ corresponding to around 2.5×10^8 cells/ml with a multiplicity of infection of 20 (ratio of phage to cells) (see **Note 9**).

4. After 60–90 min of incubation with the helper phage add 70 µg/ml kanamycin (or appropriate antibiotic depending on the chosen helper phage) to the culture, and continue the incubation with shaking for an additional 5 h.

5. Discard the bacteria by centrifuging at $3800 \times g$ for 20 min at 4 °C.

6. Recover the supernatant and repeat the centrifugation to discard residual bacteria.

7. Dissolve 40 g/l PEG 8000 and 30 g/l NaCl in the recovered supernatant and incubate it for 1 h on ice.

8. Spin down the phage by centrifuging at $15,000 \times g$ for 30 min, carefully discard the supernatant, and resuspend each pellet in 6 ml 10 mM Tris–HCl, pH 8.5.

9. Collect phage suspensions in 85 ml centrifuge tubes, two suspensions in each tube and centrifuge at $3800 \times g$ for 5 min at 4 °C to get rid of any bacterial residue. Transfer the supernatant to a fresh bottle.

10. Denaturation of the phage protein: add two volumes of PPB2 buffer to the phage suspension and swirl gently, then incubate the mixture at room temperature for 3 min, then add 1.5 volumes of PPB3, gently mix the solution by inversion and incubate in ice-cold water for 10 min.

11. Centrifuge at $16,500 \times g$ for 30 min at 4 °C, decant the supernatant to a fresh bottle and add at least two volumes of 100 % ethanol. Incubate for 1 h in ice-cold water.

12. Centrifuge at $16,500 \times g$ for 30 min at 4 °C and wash the obtained single-stranded DNA (pellet) first with 70 % ethanol, followed by repelleting by centrifugation then a final wash with

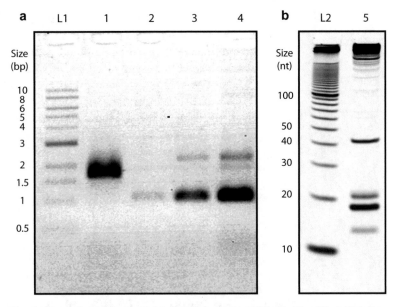

Fig. 3 Helper phage strategy. (**a**) 1.5% agarose gel (MgCl₂ 10 mM): 1 kb ladder (*L1*); M13 DNA control (*lane 1*); single-stranded phagemid DNA at 50, 250, and 500 ng/µl (*lanes 2, 3*, and *4*, respectively). (**b**) Denaturing PAGE (14%) of digested phagemid DNA containing a "crystal pseudogene" [9]

100% ethanol. Remove the ethanol and leave the tube containing the DNA pellet on the bench to dry (*see* **Note 10**).

13. Resuspend each pellet in 1 ml of 10 mM Tris–HCl (pH 8–8.5) and analyze the DNA on 2% agarose gel, running for 3 h at 70 V (Fig. 3a) (*see* **Notes 11, 12** and **13**).

14. Hairpin digestion: Digest 30–50 ng/µl phagemid DNA in 1× Tango buffer using 1 U/µl of BseGI restriction enzyme (the digestion can be performed in 50 µl in a PCR tubes for pilot experiments or in a 1.5 ml Eppendorf tube with bigger volumes depending on the amount of DNA oligonucleotides needed. Incubate the reaction mixture at 55 °C overnight.

15. Digestion products are loaded on a denaturing polyacrylamide following the same procedure described above in paragraph Subheading 3.2 (Fig. 3b) (*see* **Note 8**).

4 Notes

1. The pseudogene could be created directly by using MOSIC pseudogene calculator software on Högberg group webpage: http://www.hogberglab.net/software/. It is enough to insert a list of the desired oligonucleotides and the pseudogene sequence will be automatically provided, ready to be ordered.

2. It is convenient to order the pseudogene from the gene synthesis company directly in a vector containing fl origin of replication (for helper phage strategy) and it is important to ask for directional cloning (this will make sure that the helper phage will pack the right strand containing the pseudogene sequence). Note that for one common phagemid, those based on pBluescript, the wording in the literature can be confusing. In the ones based on pBluescriptII(+), these phagemids have the sense strand of the β-galactosidase gene secreted within the phage particles. It should be noted however, that the sense strand of this β-galactosidase gene is actually the antisense strand of the vector. So for pBluescriptII(+) and derived vectors, the pseudogene should be encoded in reverse complement on the gene map (normally this means having the 5′ of the pseudogene to the T3 promoter).

3. Linearization of the pseudogene has to be performed by using non-palindromic sequences such as BsaI-HF (reported here) or BsmBI (CGTCTC), this is to prevent the formation of pseudogene concatemers containing positive and negative strands on the same side during the ligation step.

4. It is crucial that the nicked strand is that one containing the desired oligonucleotide sequences.

5. Double nicking site on the pseudogene is not mandatory but it seems to increase the efficiency of phi29 DNA polymerase to start Amplification (RCA).

6. The concentration of T4 gene 32 can be increased up to 0.25 µg/µl to exclude any traces of double-stranded DNA.

7. Recently it has been experienced that an extra desalting step by using D-Tube dialyzer (Millipore) on RCA products increases the performance of BseGI restriction enzyme.

8. Extra bands (undigested products) could suggest that hairpin digestion requires a higher concentration of BseGI restriction enzyme or more diluted DNA in the digestion reaction. The digestion of single-stranded phagemid DNA usually provides high molecular weight bands which most likely come from the vector (Fig. 3b).

9. Helper phage can be easily amplified in JM109 *E. coli* bacteria, harvested, aliquoted and stored at –20 °C. An accurate phage titer is very crucial for achieving a high yield rescue of clean phagemid vector. This can be measured by using a standard phage titering protocol.

10. Make sure to wash the walls of the tube where the DNA can stick to improve recovery yield.

11. As a precaution the ethanol washes can be saved until the recovered DNA has been resuspended in the Tris–HCl solution and quantitated to ensure no DNA is lost in the washing steps.

12. It is convenient to load several dilutions of the resuspended pellet since the DNA is usually very concentrated. Also, about 1 in 20 molecules are usually longer contaminants from the helper phage DNA.

13. It is good practice to place the gel tank into ice-cold water (or run in a cold room) during the electrophoresis with agarose gels with $MgCl_2$, since the gels normally run hot otherwise.

Acknowledgement

We thank David and Astrid Hagelén Foundation and Svenska Sällskapet för Medicinsk Forskning (SSMF) for funding of CD; Vetenskapsrådet (Grant 2013-5883) and Stiftelsen för Strategisk Forskning (SSF, grant FFL12-0219) to B.H. Funding for open access charge: Vetenskapsrådet (Swedish Research Council).

References

1. Merrifield RB (1963) Solid phase peptide synthesis. I. Synthesis of a tetrapeptide. J Am Chem Soc 85(14):2149–2154. doi:10.1021/Ja00897a025

2. Badi N, Lutz JF (2009) Sequence control in polymer synthesis. Chem Soc Rev 38(12):3383–3390. doi:10.1039/B806413j

3. Oberacher H, Niederstatter H, Parson W (2005) Characterization of synthetic nucleic acids by electrospray ionization quadrupole time-of-flight mass spectrometry. J Mass Spectrom 40(7):932–945. doi:10.1002/Jms.870

4. Semenyuk A, Ahnfelt M, Nilsson CE, Hao XY, Foldesi A, Kao YS, Chen HH, Kao WC, Peck K, Kwiatkowski M (2006) Cartridge-based high-throughput purification of oligonucleotides for reliable oligonucleotide arrays. Anal Biochem 356(1):132–141. doi:10.1016/J.Ab.2006.05.008

5. Zhang DY, Turberfield AJ, Yurke B, Winfree E (2007) Engineering entropy-driven reactions and networks catalyzed by DNA. Science 318(5853):1121–1125.doi:10.1126/science.1148532

6. Kosuri S, Eroshenko N, LeProust EM, Super M, Way J, Li JB, Church GM (2010) Scalable gene synthesis by selective amplification of DNA pools from high-fidelity microchips. Nat Biotechnol 28(12):1295. doi:10.1038/Nbt.1716

7. Sha RJ, Birktoft JJ, Nguyen N, Chandrasekaran AR, Zheng JP, Zhao XS, Mao CD, Seeman NC (2013) Self-assembled DNA crystals: the impact on resolution of 5 '-phosphates and the DNA source. Nano Lett 13(2):793–797. doi:10.1021/Nl304550c

8. Lohmann JS, Stougaard M, Koch J (2007) A new enzymatic route for production of long 5 '-phosphorylated oligonucleotides using suicide cassettes and rolling circle DNA synthesis. BMC Biotechnol 7:49. doi:10.1186/1472-6750-7-49

9. Ducani C, Kaul C, Moche M, Shih WM, Hogberg B (2013) Enzymatic production of 'monoclonal stoichiometric' single-stranded DNA oligonucleotides. Nat Methods 10(7):647–652. doi:10.1038/Nmeth.2503

10. Ducani C, Bernardinelli G, Hogberg B (2014) Rolling circle replication requires single-stranded DNA binding protein to avoid termination and production of double-stranded DNA. Nucleic Acids Res 42(16):10596–10604. doi:10.1093/Nar/Gku737

Chapter 8

Rapid Assembly of DNA via Ligase Cycling Reaction (LCR)

Sunil Chandran

Abstract

The assembly of multiple DNA parts into a larger DNA construct is a requirement in most synthetic biology laboratories. Here we describe a method for the efficient, high-throughput, assembly of DNA utilizing the ligase chain reaction (LCR). The LCR method utilizes non-overlapping DNA parts that are ligated together with the guidance of bridging oligos. Using this method, we have successfully assembled up to 20 DNA parts in a single reaction or DNA constructs up to 26 kb in size.

Key words Synthetic biology, DNA assembly, High-throughput, Ligase chain reaction, LCR

1 Introduction

The assembly of DNA parts into larger DNA assemblies is a routine operation in most synthetic biology laboratories. DNA constructs, typically 3–20 kb in length and consisting of 2–12 DNA parts, can be assembled and introduced into strains for various purposes. While numerous DNA assembly methods are currently available [1, 2], they are all limited in the number of DNA parts that can be assembled, or have inconvenient assemblies, or are not amenable to high-throughput operations. The ligase cycling reaction (LCR) method on the other hand enables the assembly of a large number of DNA parts via an automatable workflow in a very short amount of time. LCR assembly is unique among DNA assembly methods because DNA constructs (stitches) are built from non-overlapping DNA parts (mules) using bridging oligonucleotides to guide assembly. LCR assembly utilizes single-stranded bridging oligonucleotides complementary to the ends of the DNA parts to be assembled (Fig. 1). After an initial denaturation at high temperature, the upper (or lower) strands of neighboring DNA parts anneal at lower temperature on both "halves" of the provided bridging oligo after which a thermostable ligase joins the DNA backbones via a phosphodiester bond without introducing any scar sequences. In

Randall A. Hughes (ed.), *Synthetic DNA: Methods and Protocols*, Methods in Molecular Biology, vol. 1472,
DOI 10.1007/978-1-4939-6343-0_8, © Springer Science+Business Media New York 2017

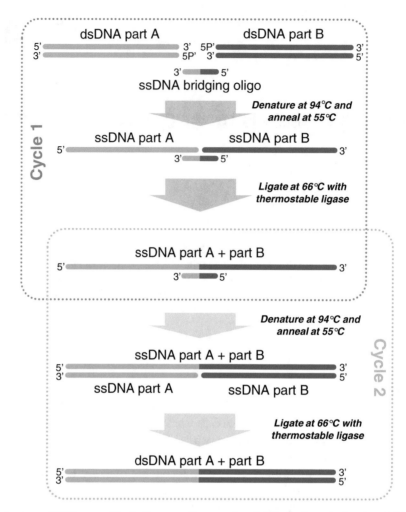

Fig. 1 Mechanism of DNA assembly via ligase cycling reaction (LCR). Custom single-stranded bridging oligos complementary to the ends of neighboring DNA parts serve as a template to bring the upper strands of denatured (5′-phosphorylated) DNA parts together, after which a thermostable ligase joins the DNA backbones. In the second and subsequent temperature cycles, the assembled upper strand serves as a template for ligation of the lower strand. Typically, 50 denaturation-annealing-ligation temperature cycles are used for the assembly of many DNA parts into complex DNA constructs

subsequent denaturation-annealing-ligation temperature cycles, the assembled upper (or lower) strand serves as a template for assembly of the lower (or upper) strand. By applying multiple temperature cycles, many DNA parts can be assembled into complex DNA constructs. Using the method outlined below, we have managed to successfully assemble DNA constructs up to 26 kb in length using 20 DNA parts [3] (*see* **Note 1**).

2 Materials

2.1 Reagents for DNA Part Amplification, Purification, and Assembly

1. Phusion Hot-Start Flex DNA Polymerase with supplied 10× buffer and dNTPs (New England Biolabs).

2. T4 polynucleotide kinase (New England Biolabs).

3. DpnI (New England Biolabs).

4. AxyPrep Mag PCR clean-up kit (Axygen Scientific) or similar.

5. Ampligase Thermostable DNA ligase and buffer (Epicentre Biotechnologies).

6. 8 % v/v DMSO.

7. 0.45 M Betaine (Fluka 14290).

8. XL1-Blue chemically competent *E. coli* cells.

9. TransforMax EPI300 electrocompetent *E. coli* cells (Epicentre Biotechnologies) or similar high-efficiency competent strain.

10. Commercially synthesized oligonucleotides.

11. 0.2 mL Thin-walled PCR tubes.

12. 1.5 mL Microcentrifuge tubes.

13. Agarose gel: Agarose Molecular Biology Grade (Fisher part number BP1356-100). Place gel trays into the casting tray, and place the comb of your choice into the slot in the gel tray. Add 1 g of agarose to a clean 250 mL bottle or flask. Add 100 mL 1× TAE Buffer Microwave until dissolved. Allow to cool to approximately 65 °C. Add 5 μL ethidium bromide solution. Swirl, carefully, keeping bottle top or neck of flask pointed away from you. Pour (100 mL ≈ two 7 cm × 10 cm gels). After the gel has hardened, remove comb and store in 1× TAE bath, at room temperature, for up to 7 days.

14. 1× TE buffer: 10 mM Tris–HCl pH 8.0, 1 mM EDTA.

15. LB broth: Use LB broth (powdered) (Fisher P/N BP1426 or similar). Add 900 mL of dH_2O to a clean 1 L flask or bottle. Add 25 g of LB broth to the flask or bottle. Stir until powder is dissolved. Transfer the solution to a 1 L graduated cylinder and add DiH_2O until the total volume of 1 L is reached. Transfer the solution to a glass media bottle. Loosely cap and sterilize by autoclaving for 20 min at 15 psi (1.05 kg/cm^2) on liquid cycle.

2.2 Equipment

1. Thermocycler.

2. Fragment Analyzer (optional).

3. Agarose gel electrophoresis equipment (gel rigs, casting trays, combs).

4. Bacterial cultivation equipment (shakers, incubators).

5. Spectrophotometer (Nanodrop or similar).

3   Methods

3.1   Design of Bridging Oligos

1. Design flanking primers to amplify all of the desired parts to be assembled from genomic DNA or purified plasmids (*see* **Note 2**).

2. Design half-bridging oligonucleotides with a target melting temperature (T_m) of 70 °C under LCR assembly conditions (i.e., 50 mM monovalent anions, 10 mM divalent anions, and 3 nM DNA) and subsequently combine the two-half sequences into a complete bridging oligonucleotide spanning across the two DNA parts (*see* **Note 3**).

3. Order desalted bridging oligonucleotides from a commercial oligonucleotide supplier.

3.2   Preparation of DNA Parts for Assembly

1. Set up PCR reactions to amplify all of the component parts to perform the assembly as per the Phusion DNA polymerase supplier-recommended conditions (https://www.neb.com/protocols/1/01/01/pcr-protocol-m0530). In general, in a 0.2 mL PCR tube add 10–100 ng of template DNA, 1× Phusion Hot-Start Flex buffer, 200 µM dNTPs, 0.5 µM forward primer, 0.5 µM reverse primer, 1 unit of Phusion Hot-Start Flex DNA polymerase, and water to a final volume of 50 µL.

2. Amplify each DNA part using the conditions recommended by the Phusion DNA polymerase supplier (e.g., https://www.neb.com/protocols/1/01/01/pcr-protocol-m0530). Adjust the annealing and extension conditions specific to the primers and lengths specific to each DNA part. In general, use the following temperature cycles: 1 cycle of 30 s at 98 °C; 30 cycles of denaturation at 98 °C for 10 s, annealing for 30 s at a temperature specific to the primers T_m (preferably between 55 and 60 °C), and extension at 72 °C for a time period specific to the length of each DNA part (15–30 s extension time per kb of DNA); 1 cycle of 4 min at 72 °C; incubation at 4 °C till the samples are analyzed.

3. Verify the successful amplification of the component parts by running a 5 µL aliquot of each PCR on a 1% agarose gel. Visualize the gel on a transilluminator or gel-imaging system.

4. If plasmid DNA is used as the template to amplify a component part, treat with DpnI as follows to remove the plasmid DNA template. To a 50 µL PCR reaction generated above add 20 U DpnI followed by incubation for 60 min at 37 °C and 20 min at 65 °C to degrade the methylated plasmid DNA.

5. Purify the PCR-amplified DNA parts using the AxyPrep Mag PCR clean-up kit (or similar PCR clean-up kit) according to the manufacturer's instructions. Purify 150 µL worth of PCR reaction mixture and concentrate the sample by eluting into 45 µL 1× TE buffer.

6. Analyze the DNA parts for the correct fragment size and purity using capillary electrophoresis on a fragment analyzer or by agarose gel electrophoresis. Measure the DNA concentrations using a spectrophotometer.

7. Following the purification and quantification, prepare a 20 µL reaction mixture in a 0.2 mL thin-walled PCR tube containing 90 fmol of each purified DNA part, 5 mM ATP, and 10 U T4 polynucleotide kinase in 1× Ampligase thermostable DNA ligase reaction buffer (*see* **Note 4**).

8. Incubate the reaction for 1 h at 37 °C followed by 20 min at 65 °C in a thermocycler. This reaction can be used directly in the subsequent assembly reaction with no further treatment.

3.3 DNA Assembly via Ligase Cycling Reaction

1. To the reaction mixture from above in a thin-walled PCR tube (Subheading 3.2, **step 8**), add 0.3 units/mL Ampligase Thermostable DNA ligase.

2. Add bridging oligonucleotides to a final concentration of 30 nM.

3. Add DMSO (8 % v/v final) and 0.45 M betaine (0.45 M final) to the reaction.

4. Add 1× Ampligase thermostable DNA ligase reaction buffer to bring up the volume to 25 µL.

5. Place tube in thermocycler and run the following temperature cycle: 2 min 94 °C and 50 cycles of 10 s 94 °C, 30 s 55 °C, and 60 s 66 °C, followed by incubation at 4 °C.

3.4 Transformation to E. coli, Colony Counting, and Restriction Endonuclease DNA Fragment Analysis

1. After DNA assembly, transform a 2.5 µL aliquot of the reaction mixture into 40 µL XL1-Blue chemically competent *E. coli* cells (3–5×10^7 CFUs/µg pUC19) or 40 µL TransforMax EPI300 electrocompetent *E. coli* cells (10^9–10^{10} CFUs/µg pUC19), according to the manufacturer's instructions (*see* **Note 5**).

2. After transformation, dilute the cells in Luria Broth (LB) and plate on LB agar plates containing 100 µg/mL carbenicillin.

3. After overnight incubation at 37 °C, count the colony-forming units (CFUs). Pick colonies (up to 30 per assembly reaction, if available) into liquid LB medium containing 100 µg/mL carbenicillin.

4. Shake overnight at 37 °C and isolate the plasmids via standard miniprep protocols and analyze via sequencing or restriction digest analysis for the correct clone.

4 Notes

1. As with any assembly method, the efficiency of the LCR assembly method tends to drop as the number of DNA parts or the size of the entire construct increases. This method has been successfully

utilized to assemble up to 20 DNA parts (0.5 kb each) and up to 26.2 kb of DNA (six DNA parts of 4 kb each with a 2.2 kb vector). Additionally, the method outlined above works best when the DNA parts being assembled are within the 0.5–2.0 kb range. It has not yet been optimized for assembly reactions where the DNA parts vary more significantly in their sizes.

2. Amplification oligonucleotides should be 25–30 bp long and have a T_m of 60 °C for best results.

3. The simplest procedure to design an amplification or bridging oligo is to copy 25–30 bp of the start or end of the DNA part (making sure that the oligo ends in a G or a C, and analyzing the T_m using a variety of online tools or user-specific software.

4. DNA has a molecular weight of ca. 630 g/mol/bp. Per 1000 bp, 90 fmol equals 57 ng.

5. While the method outlined above has been optimized to construct DNA constructs up to 26.2 kb, larger DNA constructs should be possible with an *E. coli* strain that can maintain larger DNA plasmids.

Acknowledgements

This work was funded by Defense Advanced Research Projects Agency (DARPA) Living Foundries grant HR001-12-3-0006.

References

1. Ellis T, Adie T, Baldwin GS (2011) DNA assembly for synthetic biology: from parts to pathways and beyond. Integr Biol 3:109–118

2. Merryman C, Gibson DG (2012) Methods and applications for assembling large DNA constructs. Metab Eng 14:196–204

3. de Kok S, Stanton LH, Slaby T, Durot M, Holmes VF, Patel KG, Platt D, Shapland EB, Serber Z, Dean J et al (2014) Rapid and reliable DNA assembly via ligase cycling reaction. ACS Synth Biol 3:97–106

Chapter 9

PaperClip: A Simple Method for Flexible Multi-Part DNA Assembly

Maryia Trubitsyna, Chao-Kuo Liu, Alejandro Salinas, Alistair Elfick, and Christopher E. French

Abstract

Joining DNA sequences to create linear and circular constructs is a basic requirement in molecular biology. Here we describe PaperClip, a recently developed method, which enables assembly of multiple DNA sequences in one reaction in a combinatorial manner. In contrast to other homology-based multi-part assembly methods currently available, PaperClip allows assembly of a given set of parts in any order without requiring specific single-use oligonucleotides for each assembly order.

Key words Molecular cloning, DNA assembly, Single-pot assembly, Oligonucleotide annealing, Ligation, PAGE, PCR, Agarose gel electrophoresis, CPEC, SLiCE, Cell extract, Selection

1 Introduction

Cutting and re-joining of DNA sequences became possible in the early 1970s, after the discovery of restriction endonucleases [1, 2] and DNA ligase [3]. Over the subsequent decades, molecular cloning techniques have evolved to enable researchers to join DNA 'parts' together faster and more efficiently. Current DNA assembly methods can be generally divided into restriction-based methods such as Golden Gate [4], MoClo [5], BioBrick™ [6], MODAL [7], and others, and homology-based methods including Gibson assembly [8], CPEC [9], and SLiCE [10]. Generally, restriction-based methods rely on sticky ends generated by restriction endonucleases, and parts must therefore be free of certain "forbidden" restriction sites. On the other hand, homology-based methods rely on homology between the ends of the parts to be assembled; hence, parts must be remade (e.g., by PCR), if they are to be assembled in a different order, and each assembly therefore requires multiple unique single-use oligonucleotides. This becomes expensive and inconvenient if many different assemblies are to be made from a set of parts.

Randall A. Hughes (ed.), *Synthetic DNA: Methods and Protocols*, Methods in Molecular Biology, vol. 1472, DOI 10.1007/978-1-4939-6343-0_9, © Springer Science+Business Media New York 2017

PaperClip DNA assembly [11] is a homology-based method, and does not involve use of restriction enzymes, and thus does not require mutagenesis of forbidden restriction sites. Like other homology-based methods, PaperClip allows construction of multi-part plasmids in a single reaction; however, in contrast to other methods, it allows assembly of a set of parts in multiple different orders without the requirement for order-specific oligonucleotides, saving time and money. While PaperClip assembly is directed by oligonucleotides, these are general in nature, and the same oligonucleotides can be used for any assembly involving a given part, regardless of which other parts are upstream or downstream of it. Another key feature of PaperClip assembly is that parts may be introduced into the assembly reaction in various different forms, including linear PCR products, linearized plasmids containing the desired part sequence, or circular plasmids bearing the desired part. This provides speed and flexibility, allowing immediate use of existing part libraries cloned in any format, in contrast to some other methods, which require parts to be cloned in specific donor plasmids.

To summarize the procedure: for each part to be used in PaperClip assembly, four oligonucleotides, each around 40 bases in length, should be obtained: two (forward and reverse) matching the upstream end, and two (forward and reverse) matching the downstream end of the sequence which is to become the part (Fig. 1a).

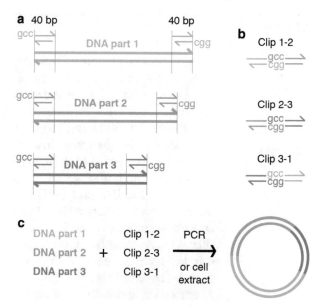

Fig. 1 Scheme of the PaperClip assembly method. (**a**) For each DNA part to be joined, four oligonucleotides of ~40 bp should be obtained. The upstream half-clip contains a GCC sticky end, and the downstream half-clip contains a compatible GGC sticky end. (**b**) After phosphorylation and annealing of oligonucleotides they are ligated in pairs according to the desired order of the DNA parts in the final construct, creating full clips. (**c**) Clips guide the order of DNA parts during PCR or cell extract-mediated assembly

These are annealed in pairs to generate two double-stranded DNA "half-clips," the upstream half-clip and downstream half-clip, corresponding to the two ends of the part. Each half-clip bears a three-base 5′ overhang at its outer end: GCC at the upstream end, and GGC at the downstream end. These half-clips can be stored with the part and may be used in any assembly involving this part.

For each join to be made in an assembly, the downstream half-clip of one part is ligated to the upstream half-clip of the next part, generating a full clip (Fig. 1b). These clips will guide the DNA parts to join in the desired order during PCR or cell extract-mediated assembly (Fig. 1c). Since all the half-clips have identical sticky ends, any part can be joined with any other part, guided by the corresponding full clips. When creating fusion proteins, the GCC scar between parts will be transcribed as alanine, a small amino acid residue, which in most cases does not interfere with protein folding and function. In our laboratory, to date, up to eight parts have been successfully assembled in a single reaction, creating plasmids up to 7.4 kb in size.

In addition to simply joining existing part sequences, it is also possible to add tags, linkers, or any other short intervening sequences between any two parts during assembly. This is accomplished by preparing the sequence to be inserted in the form of four overlapping oligonucleotides, which are ligated with the clip oligonucleotides prior to assembly (Fig. 2) to generate a clip containing the desired insertion.

Optionally, parts may be amplified by PCR prior to assembly, using the upstream forward and downstream reverse clip oligonucleotides (Fig. 3) as primers. This is not essential; as noted below,

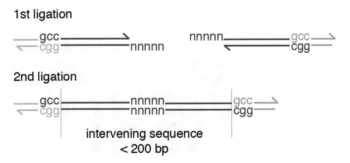

Fig. 2 Intervening sequences of 35–200 bp can be inserted between the DNA parts. These can be protein tags, linkers, etc. The intervening sequence should be obtained in the form of four oligonucleotides. After phosphorylation and annealing, the upstream half of the intervening sequence is ligated to the downstream half-clip of the preceding DNA part, and the downstream half of the intervening sequence is ligated to the upstream half-clip of the next DNA part. After 1-h incubation, the contents of the two ligations are mixed together and the intervening sequence is restored by ligation of the 5 bp sticky ends, thus creating an expanded clip including the inserted sequence

DNA part example:

5' tccggcaaaaaagggcaaggtgtcaccaccctgccctttttctttaaaaccgaaaagattacttcgcgtt
atgcaggcttcctcgctcactgactcgctgcgctcggtcgttcggctgcggcgagcggtatcagctcactca
aaggcggtaatacggttatccacagaatcaggggataacgcaggaaagaacatgtgagcaaaagg
ccagcaaaaggccaggaaccgtaaaaaggccgcgttgctggcgtttttccacaggctccgcccccctg
acgagcatcacaaaaatcgacgctcaagtcagaggtggcgaaacccgacaggactataaagatacc
aggcgtttccccctggaagctccctcgtgcgctctcctgttccgaccctgccgcttaccggatacctgtccg
cctttctcccttcgggaagcgtggcgctttctcatagctcacgctgtaggtatctcagttcggtgtaggtcgttc
gctccaagctgggctgtgtgcacgaacccccccgttcagcccgaccgctgcgccttatccggtaactatcg
tcttgagtccaacccggtaagacacgacttatcgccactggcagcagccactggtaacaggattagcag
agcgaggtatgtaggcggtgctacagagttcttgaagtggtggcctaactacggctacactagaagaac
agtatttggtatctgcgctctgctgaagccagttaccttcggaaaaagagttggtagctcttgatccggcaaa
caaaccaccgctggtagcggtggttttttg 3'

Upstream Forward (UF)
GCCtccggcaaaaaagggcaaggtgtcaccaccctgccctttttc

Upstream Reverse (UR)
aaagggcagggtggtgacaccttgccctttttgccgga

Downstream Forward (DF)
tccggcaaacaaaccaccgctggtagcggtggtttttttg

Downstream Reverse (DR)
GGCcaaaaaaaccaccgctaccagcggtggtttgtttgcc

Fig. 3 An example of oligonucleotide design for PaperClip. The upstream forward is the first 40 bases plus GCC at the 5′ end. The upstream reverse is the reverse complement of the first 37 bases. The downstream forward is the last 40 bases of the DNA part. The downstream reverse is the reverse complement of the last 37 bases plus GGC at the 5′ end

parts can also be introduced into the assembly reaction in the form of pre-existing plasmids, provided that the antibiotic resistance marker on the part plasmids is different to that used to select the final assembled product.

The overall workflow for PaperClip assembly is therefore as follows (Fig. 4):

For each part in the library:

- Design and obtain clip oligonucleotides.
- Anneal and phosphorylate oligonucleotides to generate half-clips for each part. These may be stored with the part and used in any future assembly involving that part.

For each assembly to be made:

- Ligate half-clips (optionally inserting new sequences between) to form clips.

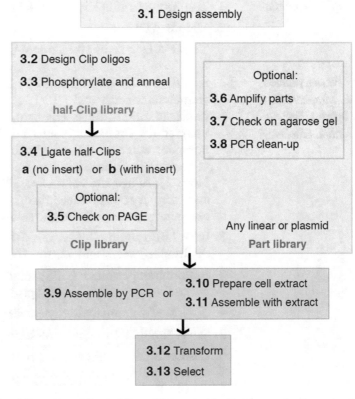

Fig. 4 Overall workflow of PaperClip assembly. Numbers refer to protocols in Subheading 3 of this chapter

- (Optional) Test ligation by SDS-PAGE.
- (Optional) Amplify parts by PCR prior to assembly.
- Conduct the assembly reaction using clips and parts. This may be done either by cell-extract-mediated recombination (as in SLiCE) or by PCR (as in CPEC).
  Transform competent cells and select for correct assembly.

2 Materials

Prepare all solutions using ultrapure water, at room temperature. Keep all stocks containing DNA on ice when in use. Store DNA stocks at −20 °C. General materials required are 1.5 ml microcentrifuge tubes, 0.2 ml clear PCR tubes, centrifuge, ice, pipettes and tips, nuclease-free water (e.g., Qiagen), ultrapure water, magnetic stirrer, water bath, heat block, and thermal cycler or incubator to be used at 16, 37, and 65 °C and for slow cooling from 95 °C to room temperature (*see* **Note 1**).

2.1 Clip Preparation

1. T4 polynucleotide kinase (PNK) and 10× buffer for T4 PNK.
2. 10 mM ATP.
3. T4 DNA ligase and 10× T4 DNA ligase buffer.

2.2 Polyacrylamide Gel Electrophoresis (for Optional Testing of Ligation Efficiency)

1. 5× TBE buffer: 1.1 M Tris, 900 mM borate, 25 mM ethylene-diaminetetraacetic acid (EDTA), pH 8.3. Weigh 2.34 g of disodium EDTA, 27 g Tris base, and 13.75 g of boric acid. Place all the components into a 600 ml glass beaker and add ultrapure water to 375 ml. While mixing the solution with a magnetic stirrer, adjust pH to 8.3 with concentrated HCl (*see* **Note 2**). Adjust the volume to 500 ml with ultrapure water, and store at room temperature in a closed bottle. If a white precipitate occurs, discard the solution.
2. 0.5× TBE running buffer: mix 50 ml of 5× TBE with 450 ml of ultrapure water, and store at room temperature.
3. Ammonium persulfate (APS) solution: 10 % (w/v) solution in water. Store at −20 °C in 200 μl aliquots.
4. *N,N,N,N′*-tetramethyl-ethylenediamine (TEMED).
5. SafeWhite™ DNA stain (NBS Biologicals) (*see* **Note 3**).
6. Casting module, thin and 1.0 mm spacer glass plates, 1.0 mm casting combs, buffer tank and lid, running module (for example Bio-Rad Mini-PROTEAN).
7. Electrophoresis power supply.
8. UV transilluminator.

2.3 PCR and PCR Cleanup (for Optional Amplification of Parts Prior to Assembly)

1. Thermal cycler.
2. KOD Hot Start DNA polymerase (*see* **Note 4**), 10× PCR buffer, 2 mM dNTPs, 25 mM $MgSO_4$ (Novagen).
3. 10 μM forward and reverse primers (components of the clips can be used, *see* Subheading 3.6, **step 3**).
4. Binding buffer: 5 M Gu-HCl, 30 % isopropanol.
5. Wash buffer: 10 mM Tris–HCl pH 7.5, 80 % ethanol.
6. Nuclease-free water pre-warmed to 70 °C.
7. Zymo-Spin™ IC column.

2.4 Agarose Gel Electrophoresis (for Testing of Optional PCR Amplification)

1. To prepare 50× TAE buffer mix 121 g of Tris base, 28.55 ml acetic acid, and 50 ml 0.5 M EDTA (pH 8.0), add ultrapure water up to 500 ml, and stir until dissolved. Store at room temperature for up to a year.
2. To make 1× TAE buffer mix 10 ml of 50× TAE with 490 ml of ultrapure water. 1× TAE is used for preparing agarose gels and as a running buffer.
3. Agarose, molecular grade.

4. 6× Gel loading buffer (New England BioLabs): 2.5% Ficoll®-400, 10 mM EDTA, 3.3 mM Tris–HCl, 0.08% SDS, 0.02% dye 1, 0.001% dye 2, pH 8.0 at 25 °C.

5. Electrophoresis power supply.

6. UV or blue light transilluminator.

2.5   Cell Extract Preparation

(Not required if assembly is to be performed by PCR) (*see* **Note 5**)

1. *E. coli* DH10B transformed with pSC101-BAD-gbaA, encoding the Lambda Red/ET recombination functions (available from GeneBridges).

2. 2× TY medium: 1.6% (w/v) bacto-tryptone, 1% (w/v) yeast extract, 0.5% (w/v) NaCl.

3. Tetracycline: 12% (w/v) solution in 70% ethanol. Light sensitive, store at −20 °C.

4. Arabinose: 20% (w/v) solution in water, sterile.

5. Cell resuspension buffer: 0.2 mM Ethylenediaminetetraacetic acid (EDTA), 0.5 mM dithiothreitol (DTT), 0.2 mM phenyl-methylsulfonyl fluoride (PMSF) [12]. Store at 4 °C for up to a month.

6. Sonicator: Bioruptor®Pico or similar.

7. Refrigerated centrifuge.

8. Eppendorf® Protein LoBind tubes, 0.5 ml, for storing cell extracts (*see* **Note 6**).

9. 10× Cell extract assembly buffer: 500 mM Tris pH 7.5, 100 mM $MgCl_2$, 10 mM ATP, 10 mM DTT [10].

2.6   Assembly by PCR (Not Required if Assembly Is to Be Performed with Cell Extracts)

1. Thermal cycler.

2. KOD Hot Start DNA polymerase (*see* **Note 4** and **Note 7**), 10× PCR buffer, 2 mM dNTPs, 25 mM $MgSO_4$ (Novagen).

2.7   Bacterial Transformation

1. Chemically competent cells of *E. coli* DH10B in 100 μl aliquots (*see* **Note 8**).

2. Water bath or heat block at 42 °C.

3. Recovery medium SOC: 2% (w/v) tryptone, 0.5% (w/v) yeast extract, 10 mM NaCl, 2.5 mM KCl, 10 mM $MgCl_2$, 20 mM glucose.

4. Shaker at 37 °C.

5. LB agar plates containing appropriate antibiotic and/or selection compound.

3 Methods

Carry out all steps at room temperature unless otherwise stated.

3.1 General Considerations in Planning the Assembly

1. The final construct should ideally contain a selection marker such as antibiotic resistance, or a component allowing visual screening, such as a fluorescent protein expression cassette. Having a selection marker as a separate part from the origin of replication will allow easy distinction of correct clones from false-positive clones, which may occur due to circularization of the part bearing the replication origin.

2. Parts smaller than 200 bp can be ordered as oligonucleotides and be used in the assembly as intervening sequences (Fig. 2, Subheading 3.4b, **step 2**) (*see* **Note 9**).

3. In our hands, up to eight parts can be assembled and selected on a single antibiotic, giving a final plasmid exceeding 7 kb in size.

4. When designing an expression construct it can be useful to include START and STOP codons within the promoter and terminator parts, respectively, omitting these codons from the open reading frame part—this will allow creation of fusion proteins and/or addition of N- or C-terminal tags if later required.

3.2 Design of Clip Oligonucleotides

1. For each of the DNA parts, four oligonucleotides must be obtained (Fig. 3). To make the upstream forward (UF) oligonucleotide choose the first ~40 bases; the base at the 3′ end should preferably be G or C. Add GCC at the 5′ end. This is UF (*see* **Note 10**).

2. To make the upstream reverse (UR) oligonucleotide, choose the first ~37 bases (three bases shorter than the region used for UF). Create the reverse complement strand. This is UR.

3. For the downstream forward (DF) oligonucleotide, choose the last 40 bases, and check that the three bases at the 5′ end are not GCC or GGC (*see* **Note 11**). If they are not, then use this sequence as DF. If the 5′ terminal bases are GCC or GGC, then choose the last 39 or 38 bases and repeat the check.

4. For the downstream reverse (DR) oligonucleotide, choose the sequence three bases shorter than DF (37 bases from the end if DF is 40 bp), create the reverse complement sequence, and add GGC at the 5′ end. This is DR.

5. Each half-clip when annealed together creates three base sticky ends facing outside of the part for ligation to generate full clips, and three base sticky ends facing inside of the part to prevent inappropriate ligation at the inner ends.

3.3 Phosphorylation and Annealing to Generate Half-Clips

1. Spin the tubes containing lyophilized oligonucleotides briefly (30 s at high speed) before opening, in case the pellet has become detached from the bottom of the tube.

2. Add nuclease-free water to obtain a final concentration of 100 μM, e.g., add 725 μl of water to 72.5 nmol of DNA. Mix the tube by flicking, and spin briefly to ensure that all liquid is at the bottom of the tube. Place the tubes on ice.

3. To phosphorylate oligonucleotides (*see* **Note 12**), add 20 μl of the forward oligonucleotide, 20 μl of the reverse oligonucleotide, 5 μl of 10× T4 polynucleotide kinase (PNK) buffer, 5 μl 10 mM ATP, and 0.5 μl of T4 PNK to a 0.2 ml clear PCR tube. Mix the tubes by flicking, and spin briefly to return all liquid to the bottom of the tube. Place the tubes in a pre-warmed PCR machine, water bath, or heat block and incubate for 30 min at 37 °C.

4. To anneal half-clips, place the tubes with phosphorylated oligonucleotides in a pre-warmed PCR machine at 95 °C. Slowly cool down the block from 95 to 4 °C using minimal ramp or 0.5 °C/s ramp if it can be set manually. If using a heat block pre-warm the block to 95 °C, insert the tubes, turn off the heat block, and let it cool down to room temperature. If using a water bath place the tubes in 95 °C water, turn off the heat, and allow it to cool down to room temperature. This step will create half-clips.

5. Transfer phosphorylated and annealed half-clips to pre-chilled 1.5 ml microcentrifuge tubes for ease of labeling and storing. Store at –20 °C. Before use, thaw thoroughly on ice and spin the tubes briefly (30 s, 2000×*g*) to ensure that all liquid is at the bottom of the tube. Keep the tubes on ice during the procedure.

3.4a Clip Ligation Without Insertion of Extra Elements Between Parts

1. One clip must be generated for each joint to be made between parts in the assembly. For each clip to be made add 4 μl of the downstream half-clip from the upstream part, 4 μl of the upstream half-clip from the downstream part, 1 μl of 10× T4 ligase buffer, 1 μl 10 mM ATP, and 0.5 μl T4 DNA ligase to a 1.5 ml microcentrifuge tube on ice. Mix the tubes by flicking, and spin briefly to return all liquid to the bottom of the tube. Incubate at 16 °C for 1 h.

2. Place the tubes in a pre-warmed heat block (or water bath) and incubate at 65 °C for 10 min to inactivate T4 DNA ligase. Spin the tubes briefly (30 s, 2000×*g*), and place on ice. Store at –20 °C. Before use, defrost thoroughly on ice and spin the tubes briefly (30 s, 2000×*g*). Keep the tubes on ice during the procedure.

3. To check the quality of the clips, analysis by polyacrylamide gel electrophoresis is recommended (*see* **Note 13**).

3.5 3.4b Clip Ligation with Insertion of Extra Elements Between Parts

1. The element to be inserted should be designed and prepared in the form of four oligonucleotides: UF, UR, DF, and DR, as indicated in Fig. 2 (*see* **Note 9**). These should be phosphorylated and annealed in pairs (UF with UR, DF with DR) as described in Subheading 3.3, to generate the upstream and downstream parts of the element to be inserted.

2. The ligation to prepare the expanded clip is conducted in two steps, as shown in Fig. 2. For the first step, add 4 μl of the downstream half-clip from the upstream part, 4 μl of the upstream part of the element to be inserted, 1 μl of 10× T4 ligase buffer, 1 μl 10 mM ATP, and 0.5 μl T4 DNA ligase to a 1.5 ml microcentrifuge tube on ice. To a second tube, add 4 μl of the upstream half-clip from the downstream part, 4 μl of the downstream part of the element to be inserted, 1 μl of 10× T4 ligase buffer, 1 μl 10 mM ATP, and 0.5 μl T4 DNA ligase. Mix the tubes by flicking, and spin briefly to return all liquid to the bottom of the tube. Incubate at 16 °C for 1 h.

3. For the second step of the ligation, mix 5 μl of the first ligation with 5 μl of the second ligation. Mix the tube, spin briefly, and incubate for a further 1 h at 16 °C.

4. Place the tubes in a pre-warmed heat block (or water bath) and incubate at 65 °C for 10 min to inactivate T4 DNA ligase. Spin the tubes briefly (30 s, $2000 \times g$), and place on ice. Store at −20 °C. Before use, defrost thoroughly on ice and spin the tubes briefly (30 s, $2000 \times g$). Keep the tubes on ice during the procedure.

5. To check the quality of the clips, analysis by polyacrylamide gel electrophoresis is recommended (*see* **Note 13**).

3.6 PAGE Analysis of Clip Ligation Efficiency (Optional but Recommended)

1. The following protocol relates to preparation and use of hand-cast PAGE gels in the Bio-Rad Mini-Protean or similar system.

2. Clean and dry the glass plates, set up the casting module, and insert the comb at an angle.

3. To prepare two 12% polyacrylamide mini gels (8.3×7.3 cm, 1.0 mm thickness) mix the components in a 50 ml tube in the following order: 5.9 ml ultrapure water, 3.7 ml 30% acrylamide:bisacrylamide (37.5:1), 2.4 ml 5× TBE, 200 μl 10% APS, and 10 μl TEMED. Mix gently, avoiding introduction of bubbles.

4. Pour the gel mixture using a 1 ml pipette and insert the comb completely. Leave to set for 30–40 min at room temperature.

5. Gels can be stored for up to 1 month at 4 °C, wrapped in tissue paper soaked with water, in a sealed bag or cling film.

6. Fit the gel in a running module according to the manufacturer's instructions. Pour the running buffer in the inner chamber to the top and in the outer chamber up to 7–10 cm. Usually

500 ml of 0.5× TBE buffer is sufficient. Carefully remove the comb and wash out the wells with running buffer using a 20 ml syringe and a needle.

7. Prepare the samples by mixing 0.5 μl of the full clip, 4.5 μl of nuclease-free water, and 1 μl of SafeWhite™.

8. Prepare the DNA ladder: 1 μl of 50 bp DNA Ladder (New England BioLabs), 4 μl of nuclease-free water, and 1 μl of SafeWhite™.

9. Load the samples using gel-loading tips. Apply 50 V for 10 min to allow the samples to enter the gel, change voltage to 100 V, and run the gel for 60–90 min.

10. Remove the gel from the glass plates, and proceed with visualization or post-staining (*see* **Note 3**).

11. Check the efficiency of ligation (*see* **Note 14**). Ideally clear bands should be present at the expected size for the full clip (around 83 bp, or larger if additional sequences have been inserted between the half-clips), with bands corresponding to the half-clips being faint or absent.

3.7 DNA Part Preparation

1. DNA parts can be used in the form of linear PCR products, DNA fragments excised from a plasmid, or linearized or circular plasmids which contain the desired part sequence, provided that such plasmids do not contain the antibiotic selection marker to be used for the final construct (*see* **Note 15**).

2. If it is desired to use linear PCR products as parts, these may be amplified from a plasmid or genomic DNA template using the UF and DR oligonucleotides as primers. The following protocol relates to preparation of such parts and may be omitted if parts are to be used in other formats (such as existing plasmids). Any standard PCR protocol may be used in place of the following.

3. Dilute UF and DR oligonucleotides 1:10 to obtain 10 μM final concentration (use 5 μl of 100 μM stock and 45 μl of nuclease-free water). Store diluted oligonucleotides at −20 °C. Before use thaw thoroughly on ice, spin the tubes briefly (30 s 2000×g), and keep on ice.

4. In a 0.2 ml clear PCR tube add 29 μl of nuclease-free water, 5 μl of 10× PCR buffer, 5 μl 2 mM dNTPs, 3 μl 25 mM MgSO4, 1 μl DNA template (~5 ng), 3 μl 10 μM UF, 3 μl 10 μM DR, and 1 μl polymerase (KOD Hot Start, Novagen). Flick the tube, spin briefly (30 s, 2000×g), and place in a PCR machine pre-warmed to 95 °C. Run the following program: 95 °C 2 min, 35 cycles—95 °C 20 s, the lowest melting temperature of two primers (or 70 °C if the lowest melting temperature is higher than 70 °C) 10 s, 70 °C 10 s/kb for <500 bp, 15 s/kb for 500–1000 bp, 20 s/kb for 1000–3000 bp, or 25 s/kb for >3000 bp. Hold at 10 °C.

3.8 Agarose Gel Separation of Amplified Parts

(Required only if parts have been amplified by PCR prior to assembly)

1. To check the success of the PCR amplification of the DNA parts prepare a 1% (w/v) agarose gel. Add 0.3 g molecular-grade agarose and 30 ml 1× TAE buffer in a glass beaker or heat-resistant bottle (*see* **Note 16**). Heat in the microwave until just starting to boil, e.g., ~30 s at max power 700 W. Swirl the bottle until the agarose is dissolved.

2. Cool the agarose to ~50 °C, swirling it occasionally, and add 3 μl of SaveView™ DNA stain for in-gel staining. Alternatively the gel can be stained after electrophoresis (*see* **Note 3**).

3. Clean the gel casting tray with water, dry, and wipe with 70% ethanol. Cover the sides of the tray with tape to prevent gel leakage. Place the casting tray on an even surface and fit the comb. Pour agarose till the gel is 3–5 mm high (*see* **Note 17**). Leave to set for at least 30 min at room temperature. Do not move the tray while the gel is setting (*see* **Note 18**).

4. Prepare the samples by mixing 5 μl of the PCR reaction with 1 μl of 6× gel loading dye.

5. Prepare DNA ladder by mixing 1 μl of the ladder (1 kb DNA Ladder or 1 kb Plus DNA ladder) with 4 μl nuclease-free water and 1 μl 6× gel loading dye.

6. Place the set agarose gel in the gel running chamber. Top up the chamber with 1× TAE till the gel is completely covered in buffer.

7. Carefully load the samples and the DNA ladder. Separate DNA at 60 V for 60 min.

8. Proceed to visualization or post-staining (*see* **Note 3**) if stain was not added to the gel prior to casting.

3.9 Purification of the DNA Parts

1. If the PCR resulted in a single band of the expected size, column purification can be used to remove primers, dNTPs, and polymerase. If several bands are obtained, either optimization of the PCR (*see* **Note 19**) or gel purification (*see* **Note 20**) can be performed.

2. For column purification, add 250 μl of the binding buffer to the remaining PCR mix (~45 μl). Mix by pipetting.

3. Transfer the whole mixture to the Zymo-Spin™ IC column. Place the column in the collection tube (a 1.5 ml microcentrifuge tube with the cap cut off.)

4. Spin the column for 1 min at 13,000 rpm ($12{,}470 \times g$) at room temperature. Discard the flow-through.

5. Add 500 μl of the washing buffer to the column. Repeat **step 4** two times to dry off the residual ethanol from the resin.

6. Pipette 20 μl of nuclease-free water pre-warmed to 70 °C directly on the resin of the column. Let stand at room temperature for 5 min.

7. Place the column in a new collection tube. Spin the column for 1 min at 13,000 rpm ($12,470 \times g$) at room temperature. This should result in ~18 μl of >100 ng/μl DNA concentration, which is enough for ~18 assemblies if the part is around 1 kb.

8. Store DNA at −20 °C. Before use defrost thoroughly on ice and spin the tubes briefly (30 s, $2000 \times g$). Keep on ice.

3.10 Assembly by PCR

1. The assembly reaction should contain 15 nM DNA parts and 300 nM clips, 200 nM dNTPs, 1.5 mM $MgSO_4$, 1× KOD Hot Start Buffer (Novagen), and 1.0 U KOD Hot Start Polymerase (Novagen) in 50 μl final volume.

2. Example of a 2-part assembly reaction: 32.6 μl nuclease-free water, 2 μl of 2 kb DNA part 1 (100 ng/μl), 1 μl of 1 kb DNA part 2 (100 ng/μl), 0.2 μl clip 1–2, 0.2 μl clip 2–1, 5 μl 2 mM dNTPs, 3 μl 25 mM $MgSO_4$, 5 μl 10× KOD Hot Start Buffer (Novagen), and 1 μl KOD Hot Start Polymerase (Novagen). Mix the tube, spin briefly (30 s, $2000 \times g$), and place in a PCR machine pre-warmed to 95 °C.

3. Run the following program: 95 °C 2 min; 20 cycles (*see* **Note 6**) of 95 °C 20 s, slow cooling down to 70 °C (minimum ramp speed, or 0.5 °C/s if this can be set manually), and 70 °C 1 min (for 3000 bp final construct; adjust as required according to the size of the construct); hold at 10 °C.

3.11 Preparation of Cell Extracts

1. In applications where PCR-based assembly is not desired (*see* **Note 5**), assemblies can be performed using in vitro recombination mediated by cell extracts (a modification of SLiCE [10]). This method is less effective than PCR based for assemblies containing more than three parts, but the size of the final product is not limited by the performance of the polymerase during PCR.

2. Use a single colony of *E. coli* DH10B freshly transformed with lambda red plasmid pSC101-BAD-gbaA (GeneBridges) to inoculate 5 ml LB medium contacting 12 μg/ml tetracycline (Tet12). Protect from light by covering in foil. Incubate for 16–20 h at 30 °C with shaking at 200 rpm.

3. Inoculate 500 ml of 2× TY Tet12 medium with 5 ml overnight culture. Cover the flask in foil and incubate at 30 °C with 200 rpm agitation until OD_{600} reaches 0.38.

4. Add 7.5 ml 20 % (w/v) arabinose (final concentration 0.3 %) to induce expression of recombination proteins. Incubate at 37 °C and 200 rpm for 45 min.

5. Transfer the culture to ice-cold centrifuge bottles. Spin down the cells at $5000 \times g$ for 20 min at 4 °C. Decant the supernatant.

6. Weigh a 1.5 ml microcentrifuge tube and transfer the pellet into it. Weigh again and calculate the pellet weight. Keep the pellet on ice at all times and minimize exposure to room temperature.

7. Resuspend the cell pellet in ice-cold cell resuspension buffer in the ratio of 1 g of pellet to 1.3 ml buffer. Proceed to sonication immediately.

8. Disrupt the cells by sonication in a pre-chilled (4 °C) chamber for 5 min using cycles 30-s ON and 30-s OFF.

9. Remove cell debris by centrifugation at $10000 \times g$ for 5 min at 4 °C.

10. Collect the supernatant and add an equal volume of sterile 100% glycerol. Store in 20 μl aliquots at –20 °C in Eppendorf® Protein LoBind 0.5 ml tubes.

3.12 Cell Extract-Mediated Assembly

1. The assembly reaction is performed in 10 μl final volume and contains 10 nM backbone, 100 nM insert, 500 nM of both clips, 1 μl of 10× cell extract buffer, and 1 μl of cell extract (*see* **Note 7**).

2. Example of reaction mixture for a 2-part assembly: 1.3 μl of 2 kb part 1 (backbone, 100 ng/μl), 6.5 μl 1 kb part 2 (insert, 100 ng/μl), 0.36 μl clip 1–2, 0.36 μl clip 2–1, 1 μl of 10× cell extract buffer, and 1 μl of cell extract. Mix by pipetting. Incubate at 37 °C for 1 h. Proceed with transformation.

3.13 Transformation

1. If the antibiotic selection cassette was introduced as part of a plasmid which can be propagated in the destination strain, DpnI digestion is recommended after the assembly and prior to transformation in order to destroy the parent plasmid and reduce the number of colonies which contain this plasmid rather than the desired construct. After the assembly reaction, add 1 μl of DpnI to 50 μl reaction and incubate for 1 h at 37 °C. Proceed with transformation as usual.

2. Add 5 μl of PCR assembly mix, or 8 μl of cell extract-mediated assembly mix, to 100 μl chemically competent cells *E. coli* DH10B thawed on ice (*see* **Note 8**). Mix the tubes gently. Avoid holding the tubes at the base, in order to minimize temperature fluctuation.

3. Incubate on ice for 30 min. Do not mix the tubes.

4. Place the tubes in a heat block or water bath pre-warmed to 42 °C for 90 s. Return the tubes to ice. Do not mix the tubes.

5. Add 400 μl SOC medium at room temperature to the transformation mixture. Mix by inverting the tubes gently.

6. Incubate the tubes on a rotary shaker at 200 rpm at 37 °C for 70–90 min.

7. Plate out 200 µl on two LB agar plates contacting the appropriate antibiotic and/or selection additives.

3.14 Selection of the Correct Clones

1. As noted above, the best results are obtained if the antibiotic selection marker is introduced as a separate DNA part from the origin of replication. If this cassette comes from a plasmid, which cannot replicate in the recipient strain, all of the final clones will be products of the assembly. For example, we routinely use a kanamycin resistance cassette carried on a plasmid containing the R6K origin of replication, and the destination strain *E. coli* DH10B, in which this plasmid cannot be propagated due to the absence of the required *pir* proteins. Thus all kanamycin-resistant clones must contain assembled plasmid DNA.

2. If the vector backbone contains a marker, which will be lost after the assembly (for example RFP, *lacZ*), then colonies containing assembled plasmids can easily be distinguished visually from those containing the vector alone.

3. Multiple antibiotic and/or color selection can be used to reduce the number of background colonies.

4. Colonies may be screened by colony PCR using the UF oligonucleotide of one part and the DR oligonucleotide of another, to check that all parts in between are present.

4   Notes

1. For clip preparation all incubation steps can be conveniently performed in a thermal cycler. Alternatively, phosphorylation can be done at 37 °C in an incubator, a water bath, or a heat block. Slow cooling down for annealing of half-clips can be performed in a water bath or a heat-block by turning it off after preheating to 95 °C. Ligation can be done at 16 °C in an incubator or a cooling water bath. Ligase inactivation at 65 °C can be done in a water bath or a heat block.

2. Adequate personal protection should be worn when handling concentrated HCl.

3. Gels can be post-stained with GelGreen™ DNA stain (Biotum, Inc). Dilute GelGreen™ stain in water according to the manufacturer's instructions (15 µl for 50 ml water). Place the gel in the staining solution, and incubate for 10–20 min protected from light. Shaking is not necessary. Proceed with visualization. Solution can be stored at room temperature, protected from light, and reused during at least 1 month.

4. Add polymerase as the last component to the PCR mix, mix the tube by flicking, spin briefly, and place the tube in a thermal cycler preheated to 95 °C.

5. Using cell extracts, up to four parts can be assembled in one reaction, though efficiency may be low for three- and four-part assemblies. This may be the method of choice to reduce the price of the assemblies or when there is some homology within the DNA sequences which may lead to deletions during PCR assembly.

6. Cell extract activity drops down with storage. Prepare small aliquots and minimize exposure of the cell extract to temperatures above –20 °C.

7. If deletions happen during PCR assembly, a reduced number of cycles might solve the problem (for example 5 cycles instead of 20). Purity of parts might also cause deletions during PCR assembly; try gel purification and re-amplification of the parts in which deletion occurred.

8. When handling competent cells, minimize their exposure to room temperature and keep them on ice. After the cells are thawed, add DNA straight away. Do not exceed 30-min incubation on ice and do not shake the tube during heat shock.

9. To design oligonucleotides for intervening sequences (Fig. 2) choose 5 bp in the middle of the sequence to be the sticky ends, which will join the two halves of the sequence. Select the 5′ half of the sequence without these 5 bp, and add GCC at the 5′ end—this is UF. Select the sequence up to and including the five central bases, and create the reverse complement—this is UR. The highlighted bases together with the 3′ half of the sequence are DF. Select the downstream end without the highlighted bases create the reverse complement and add GGC at the 5′ end—this is DR. The annealing and ligation of the intervening sequence will be efficient if it is longer than 35 bp.

10. If the position of the start and end of the DNA part is flexible, it is recommended to choose oligonucleotides with reduced ability to form hairpin structures. This can be checked at https://eu.idtdna.com/calc/analyzer.

11. It is better to avoid having a 5′ G base in the DF design to reduce formation of clip multimers during the ligation step.

12. Alternatively, the oligonucleotides may be ordered in phosphorylated form, usually at additional expense. If using prephosphorylated oligonucleotides, simply proceed with the annealing and ligation steps. It is also possible to include polynucleotide kinase in the clip ligation reactions, but this may require longer incubation periods than stated in Subheading 3.4 (e.g., overnight).

13. It is possible to use 2 % (w/v) agarose gel electrophoresis rather than PAGE to check the efficiency of ligation, but the resolution will be less than that of PAGE.

14. If less than 50 % of the DNA is ligated to create the full clips, the ligation reaction can be extended to 16 h. If there are bands of higher molecular weight than is expected for full clips (~80 bp), the ligation time can be reduced or oligonucleotides should be redesigned. Take extra care when choosing incompatible sticky ends on the inward-facing ends of the half-clips.

15. The best assembly results for high number of parts are obtained when using linear DNA parts after PCR amplification and DNA cleanup.

16. Add agarose to a dry beaker or heat-resistant bottle first, and then add 1× TAE—this will result in improved dissolution of the agarose.

17. The thinner the agarose gel, the sharper DNA bands will appear on it. The best picture can be obtained if wider wells are used with the lowest DNA sample volume (e.g., 0.75 mm × 5 mm well and 6 μl sample volume).

18. If the gel tray is moved while the agarose is setting, this will result in visible short fluorescent lines while visualizing DNA with the UV transilluminator.

19. If no bands are obtained during PCR, lower annealing temperature and a longer elongation time can be used. If the DNA part has high GC content or is long and/or amplified from the genomic DNA template, addition of DMSO to a final concentration of 2–10 % and increasing the concentration of $MgSO_4$ to 2 mM might be helpful. Change only one parameter at a time.

20. Gel purification gives the purest DNA, but usually results in low final DNA concentration. It might be useful to use a gel-purified DNA band as a template to re-amplify DNA for the assembly.

Acknowledgements

This work was supported by Engineering and Physical Sciences Research Council [EP/J02175x/1].

References

1. Arber W, Linn S (1969) DNA modification and restriction. Annu Rev Biochem 38:467–500. doi:10.1146/annurev.bi.38.070169.002343

2. Meselson M, Yuan R (1968) DNA restriction enzyme from E. coli. Nature 217(5134):1110–1114

3. Weiss B, Richardson CC (1967) Enzymatic breakage and joining of deoxyribonucleic acid, I. Repair of single-strand breaks in DNA by an enzyme system from Escherichia coli infected with T4 bacteriophage. Proc Natl Acad Sci U S A 57(4):1021–1028

4. Engler C, Kandzia R, Marillonnet S (2008) A one pot, one step, precision cloning method with high throughput capability. PLoS One 3(11), e3647. doi:10.1371/journal.pone.0003647

5. Weber E, Engler C, Gruetzner R, Werner S, Marillonnet S (2011) A modular cloning system for standardized assembly of multi-gene constructs. PLoS One 6(2), e16765. doi:10.1371/journal.pone.0016765

6. Shetty R, Lizarazo M, Rettberg R, Knight TF (2011) Assembly of BioBrick standard biological parts using three antibiotic assembly. Methods Enzymol 498:311–326. doi:10.1016/B978-0-12-385120-8.00013-9

7. Casini A, MacDonald JT, De Jonghe J, Christodoulou G, Freemont PS, Baldwin GS, Ellis T (2014) One-pot DNA construction for synthetic biology: the Modular Overlap-Directed Assembly with Linkers (MODAL) strategy. Nucleic Acids Res 42(1), e7. doi:10.1093/nar/gkt915

8. Gibson DG, Young L, Chuang RY, Venter JC, Hutchison CA 3rd, Smith HO (2009) Enzymatic assembly of DNA molecules up to several hundred kilobases. Nat Methods 6(5):343–345. doi:10.1038/nmeth.1318

9. Quan J, Tian J (2009) Circular polymerase extension cloning of complex gene libraries and pathways. PLoS One 4(7), e6441. doi:10.1371/journal.pone.0006441

10. Zhang Y, Werling U, Edelmann W (2012) SLiCE: a novel bacterial cell extract-based DNA cloning method. Nucleic Acids Res 40(8), e55. doi:10.1093/nar/gkr1288

11. Trubitsyna M, Michlewski G, Cai Y, Elfick A, French CE (2014) PaperClip: rapid multi-part DNA assembly from existing libraries. Nucleic Acids Res. doi:10.1093/nar/gku829

12. Michlewski G, Caceres JF (2010) RNase-assisted RNA chromatography. RNA 16(8):1673–1678. doi:10.1261/rna.2136010

Chapter 10

The Polymerase Step Reaction (PSR) Method for Gene and Library Synthesis

Brian S. DeDecker

Abstract

Current gene synthesis methods often incorporate a PCR-amplifying step in order to yield sufficient final product that is detectable and resolvable from multiple off-products. This amplification step can cause stochastic sampling effects that propagate errors during the synthesis and lower the variability when applied towards the construction of randomized libraries. We present the method for polymerase step reaction (PSR), a simple DNA polymerase-based gene synthesis reaction that assembles DNA oligonucleotides in a unidirectional fashion without the need for a PCR-type amplification (Lee et al., BioTechniques 59:163–166, 2015). The PSR method is simple and efficient with little off-product production, undetected stochastic sampling effects, and maximized variability when used to synthesize phage display libraries.

Key words Gene synthesis, Gene assembly, Randomized library construction, DNA polymerase, Stochastic sampling effect, Thermal cycling reaction, Variable library and single-stranded DNA

1 Introduction

As chemical synthesis is currently limited to synthesizing error-free oligonucleotides in lengths often shorter than the desired genes [1], many methods use DNA ligases or polymerases to assemble smaller purified oligonucleotide components into full-length gene products [2–4]. However, the successful assembly of the full-length sequence becomes dependent on the efficiency of a number of smaller successive reactions. The result of this approach is that the intended product may not be produced in an appreciable quantity—requiring PCR amplification to resolve the intended full-length sequence from the many incomplete and intermediate reaction products also present. Of these methods, the polymerase cycling assembly (PCA) reaction and its variations are the most widely used of the polymerase-based methods of gene synthesis [5]. As the intermediate steps and final product of PCA use PCR-type amplifications, stochastic sampling may amplify errors found in the initial oligonucleotide pools requiring a linear amplification

Randall A. Hughes (ed.), *Synthetic DNA: Methods and Protocols*, Methods in Molecular Biology, vol. 1472,
DOI 10.1007/978-1-4939-6343-0_10, © Springer Science+Business Media New York 2017

approach [6]. PCR-type steps could also compromise the construction of libraries with targeted randomization. Exponential amplification steps could reduce potential variability in the library by amplifying only a subset of the variation in the early rounds of thermal cycling. We present the alternative method of PSR [7], a polymerase-based method that assembles genes in a linear fashion without amplification that resembles solid-phase and non-polymerase-based technologies [8–11]. In PSR, a single forward primer is mixed with multiple template primers in the reverse direction (Fig. 1). Importantly, the template primers are blocked on the 3′ end, preventing their extension during thermal cycling [12]. With activity of the DNA polymerase effectively limited to the extension of the forward primer, any annealing and extension that do occur only serve to ratchet forward the construction of the primary gene product, all without amplification. This is in contrast with PCA, in which a pool of assembly primers extend in both directions to mostly generate off-products, while full-length sequence is undetectable and must be further amplified by PCR [13, 14]. Targeted variation can be incorporated within the

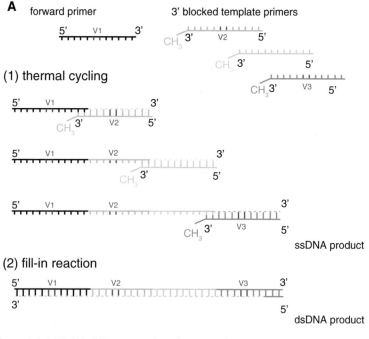

Fig. 1 (a) Schematic of PSR reaction. (*1*) Forward primer in black is mixed with a collection of successive 3′ blocked reverse direction templates. During thermal cycling the product is ratcheted forward by DNA polymerase without off-product formation or exponential amplification. The positions of three potential variable regions are shown in *red* and may be positioned anywhere within the non-overlapping regions. (*2*) The ssDNA product can be filled in with an extendable reverse primer in a second thermal cycling reaction or by other methods (*see* **Note 12**)

non-overlapping regions of the assembly primers to construct molecular libraries. After the initial thermal cycling reaction, a single-stranded DNA (ssDNA) product is produced that is still associated with some of the blocked template primers. This ssDNA PSR product can be feed into subsequent DNA polymerase-based reactions without the template primers further extending and creating more off-product. In this specific demonstration, we fill-in the ssDNA product by adding a single reverse primer (not blocked) and performing a second thermo cycling reaction. This displaces the blocked template primers and creates a double-stranded DNA product (dsDNA) that can be used in various applications.

2 Materials

Prepare all solutions using ultrapure water and analytical grade reagents. Prepare and store all reagents on ice (unless indicated otherwise).

2.1 Primer Design

1. Oligonucleotide primers: PSR works by combining one forward primer with a series of blocked template primers and performing a PCR like thermal cycling reaction with DNA polymerase [7]. The first primer is in the forward extending direction of the synthesis product while all template strands are in reverse (Fig. 1). The template primers are blocked on the 3′ end with propyl group extensions that effectively block DNA polymerase extension. Other blocking groups may be used (*see* **Note 1**). Overlapping regions between the primers are calculated for a $T_m > 64$ °C by Oligo Calc using the parameters 500 nM Primer, 50 mM salt, and the nearest-neighbor algorithm (*see* **Note 2**) [15].

For variable library synthesis, one forward primer is combined with three blocked template primers. The average length of the primers we have used is 92 bases with average overlap regions of 27 on both ends of the primer. This leaves approximately 38 bases in the middle of each primer that is free for randomizing specific positions (*see* **Note 3**).

2.2 Primer Synthesis and Purification

1. Primers (purchased from a high-quality vendor): Errors introduced during primer synthesis are the main source of errors in the final PSR product (mostly $n-1$ and $+1$ products). These errors limit the potential length of the PSR product as longer products have a reduced chance of being error free (*see* **Note 4**). Therefore, a high-quality oligonucleotide synthesis and polyacrylamide gel electrophoresis (PAGE) purification are required. For smaller primers other means of purification are possible (*see* **Note 5**).

2. Primer stock solutions: Primers are brought up to 100 μM stocks (100 pmol/μl). A typical 200 nmol primer synthesis would yield 14 nmol of PAGE-purified product to which 140 μl of PCR-grade water is added. The stock solutions are aliquoted in small batches (5–25 μl), then flash frozen in liquid nitrogen, and stored at −80 °C (*see* **Note 6**).

2.3 Reagents and Equipment

KOD Hot Start DNA Polymerase (EDM Millipore) with included buffers and reagents is used for all reactions (*see* **Note 7**).

PureLink PCR purification kit (Life Technologies) or similar.

0.2 μl Thin-walled PCR tubes.

QIAquick Gel Extraction Kit (Qiagen) or similar.

Thermocycler.

NanoDrop 2000c spectrophotometer or similar.

Agarose gel electrophoresis equipment and materials.

100 bp DNA ladder (New England Biolabs) or similar.

1 kbp DNA ladder (New England Biolabs) or similar.

3   Methods

Carry out all procedures on ice unless otherwise noted.

3.1 PSR Assembly Reaction

1. The following is mixed in a microcentrifuge tube and can be scaled up proportionally for multiple reactions. The blocked template primers have been combined for a template stock solution of 33 μM for each primer. A final ratio of 2:1 extension to template primers is used in this example, but other ratios may be better for other synthesis designs (*see* **Note 8**). The total reaction volume of 50 μl is then transferred to a thin-walled PCR tube.

Mix	Final concentration
30.5 μl Water	
3 μl DMSO	6%
3 μl 25 mM MgSO$_4$ (supplied with polymerase)	1.5 mM
5 μl 10× Buffer (supplied with polymerase)	1×
5 μl dNTP mix (2 mM each)	0.2 mM each
1 μl 100 μM Forward primer 1	2 μM
1.5 μl Primers 2–4 mix (33 μM each)	1 μM each
1 μl KOD Hot Start DNA Polymerase	

With the DNA polymerase added last and just before thermocycling.

2. The PSR reaction mix is transferred to a thermocycler with cycling conditions set as follows: 95 °C for 2 min, then 30 two-step cycles at 95 °C for 20 s and 70 °C for 2 min, followed by a 70 °C hold for 5 min. Samples are then cooled and held at 4 °C. The cycling reaction takes approximately 1.5 h (*see* **Note 9**).

3. The entire reaction is then isolated on a PureLink PCR purification column using the binding buffer included in the kit (*see* **Note 10**).

4. Yields are measured by UV absorbance on a NanoDrop 2000c spectrophotometer (Thermo Scientific) (*see* **Note 11**). For a typical reaction approximately 51 pmol of DNA is recovered giving a yield of 51% compared to the molar input of forward primer.

3.2 Complementary Strand Fill-In

1. Approximately 24% of the ssDNA from the PSR reaction (12 μl out of 50 μl) is annealed to a complementary "fill-in" primer and made double stranded with KOD polymerase. Other methods may be used to fill-in the PSR product including PCR (*see* **Note 12**). The following is mixed to a total reaction volume of 50 μl and added to thin-walled PCR tubes.

Mix	Final concentration
23.7 μl Water	
3 μl 25 mM MgSO$_4$ (supplied with polymerase)	1.5 mM
5 μl 10× Buffer (supplied with polymerase)	1×
5 μl dNTP mix (2 mM each)	0.2 mM (each)
12 μl 1 μM ssDNA from PSR rxn	0.24 μM
0.3 μl 100 μM Fill-in primer	0.6 μM
1 μl KOD Hot Start DNA Polymerase	

2. The fill-in reaction mix is transferred to a thermocycler with cycling conditions set as follows: 95 °C for 2 min, and then 25 two-step cycles at 95 °C for 20 s and 70 °C for 3 min. Samples were then cooled and held at 4 °C. The cycling reaction takes approximately 1.5 h (*see* **Note 13**). The final dsDNA product can be visualized on an agarose gel stained by ethidium bromide (*see* Fig. 2 and **Note 14**).

3. The dsDNA product is isolated by agarose gel electrophoresis (1.5%) and purified using a QIAquick Gel Extraction Kit (*see* **Note 15**). Yields are measured by UV absorbance on a NanoDrop 2000c spectrophotometer. Approximately 9.6 pmol of purified dsDNA is typically recovered from the fill-in reac-

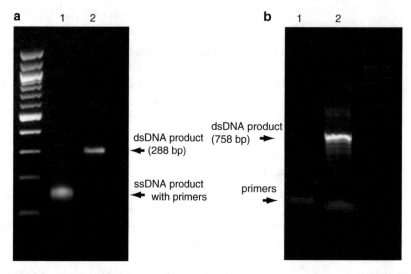

Fig. 2 (**a**) One forward primer was combined with three template primers to synthesize a 288 base pair product with three randomized sites (Fig. 1). The ssDNA PSR product with some blocked primers associated (*1*) and the filled in dsDNA product (*2*) are shown on a 1.2 % agarose gel stained with EtBr. Referenced with a 100 bp DNA ladder (New England Biolabs). Both *lanes* are prior to purification and contrary to PCA reactions, and demonstrate efficient synthesis without visible off-products. (**b**) One forward primer was combined with nine template primers to synthesize a 758 base pair product without variability. The unreacted primers (*1*) and the filled-in dsDNA product (*2*) are shown on a 1.2 % agarose gel stained with EtBr. Referenced with a 1 kb DNA ladder (New England Biolabs)

tion for a yield from this step of 78 % and a final yield of 41 % compared to the initial input amount of forward primer in the PSR reaction. PSR product with randomized regions will have mismatched bubbles present that can be removed (*see* **Note 16**). Approximately 1.0×10^{13} full-length dsDNA molecules are typically synthesized from 100 pmols of forward primer.

4   Notes

1. Other blocking groups may be used on the 3′ end of template primers to prevent DNA polymerase activity. For instance, we have also successfully used a primary amine on the 3′ end of the template stands.

2. The designed melting temperature of the overlap regions and the actual annealing temperature used during thermal cycling are variables that may be optimized. To be considered is the competition between the previous template primer fully annealed to the extending strand and the 3′ overlap region of the template primer next in line for extension.

3. If variability is not required in the synthesis product then smaller primers may be used as they would not require the

middle non-overlapping region. Primers with just two overlapping regions and no intervening sequence could be approximately 40 nucleotides long.

4. For library construction the primers need to be of the highest quality and PAGE purified. Standard error correction techniques based on mismatch repair will not work with library synthesis as the final product will inevitably have mismatched bubbles within the variable regions. We are able to obtain a low error rate of only 0.0018 per base in the final library with primers obtained from a vendor with both high-quality control for synthesis and PAGE purification. Current DNA synthesis techniques do not reach this error rate without additional purification. Typically showing coupling efficiencies of 98.5–99.5% per base, while additional synthesis errors resulting in insertions and deletions have been found to be as high as 0.5% and 0.4%, respectively [16].
The fraction of the final library population free of errors can be calculated as such.
Error rate (R), length (N), and fraction free of errors (X)

$$(1-R)^N = X$$

With an error rate of 0.0018 and a 288 base product, we find 60% of the final PSR synthesis products free of errors. For comparison, only 6% of the library pool would be error free using unpurified primers with an error rate of 0.01. The primer error rate gives an upper limit to the potential length of the final product. We predict that an 800 base pair product with the low error rate of 0.0018 would only have 24% of the final library products free of errors (mostly frame shifting).

5. More efficient HPLC-based methods of purification may work for smaller primers around 40 nucleotides long. Dual HPLC or dual PAGE should also be considered for longer final PSR products and demanding library constructions.

6. Repeated freeze thawing degraded the stock solutions of long primers, presumably due to precipitation. Aliquoting may not be needed for shorter primers that tend to be more soluble.

7. Highly processive polymerases such as KOD generate full-length product on a more consistent basis when compared to Taq and other less processive DNA polymerases.

8. We have found that many different ratios between forward and template primers will work, with 2:1 consistently giving good results. Excess forward primer increases the amount of forward product relative to the template primers and potentially reduces competition for binding sites during thermal cycling.

9. There is a competition between the extending primer and the previous template primer causing inefficiency in the forward reaction.

The forward reaction is irreversible causing the extension to ratchet forward, but the reaction still needs a repetition of thermal cycles greater than the number of template primers. Additional thermal cycles may be needed for longer PSR products using more template primers. For instance, we use 80 cycles for an approximately 750 base pair product constructed from ten primers.

10. The PureLink PCR Purification Kit specifications indicate that it is optimized to purify 100 bp to 12 kb dsDNA products. The PSR product is ssDNA, but still associated with blocked template primers. The PureLink columns will bind to this mixed stranded product and remove unbound free template primers. This purification step may not be needed as the template primers are inert and do not contribute to further off-product production in subsequent polymerase reactions. After purification, some blocked template primers still remain with the ssDNA PSR product and are competed off in subsequent fill-in reactions. If pure ssDNA is required from the PSR reaction the protocol could be modified. For example, chemistry could be added to the 5′ end of the forward primer that links it to a heat-stable resin. This would allow the associated blocked template primers to be melted off after the PSR reaction and isolating the ssDNA product.

11. When measuring the PSR reaction by UV absorbance we assume mostly dsDNA in the sample. This is only an estimate as the ssDNA PSR product is still associated with blocked template primers in an unknown ratio.

12. Other methods may be used to fill-in the PSR ssDNA product. Rather that using a fill-in primer, two separate PSR reactions designed in opposite directions can be combined to fill-in each other in a second thermocycling step. This method is similar to an overlap extension reaction with the difference being that two ssDNA PSR products are being combined, rather than two dsDNA PCR products [17, 18]. Alternatively, if a large excess of dsDNA product is needed from the PSR reaction, a PCR reaction with two end primers can be used to amplify the ssDNA PSR product. However, PCR may induce stochastic sampling errors depending on the amount of initial product from the PSR reaction.

13. The fill-in primer competes with the blocked template primers that carried through the spin column purification, thus requiring an excess of thermal cycles to fill-in the ssDNA PSR product.

14. Even with a molar excess of fill-in primer, excess single-stranded reverse direction product is not detectable on the agarose gel. Excess reverse direction ssDNA is possibly present but not detectable due to the decreased affinity ssDNA has for ethidium bromide.

15. Gel purification of the final product is not required for most applications. Much of the DNA that is purified from the dsDNA product by gel purification is blocked by template primers that will not extend in further reactions. In addition, gel purification reduces the final yield dramatically.

16. During thermal cycling the variant DNA strands will inevitably hybridize to partners that are non-complementary in the variable regions (producing mismatched bubbles). This precludes the use of methods that rely on mismatched bases for error correction. These mismatch bubbles may be resolved by cloning and transforming the library into *E. coli*. These mismatches are resolved by allowing for one round of plasmid replication and cell division before plating. A short PCR reaction is another potential method to remove mismatches in variable regions. A PCR reaction on the ssDNA PSR product with a large excess of primers and limited number of thermal cycles could complement the mismatches without excessive amplification.

Acknowledgment

This work was supported in part by a grant from the National Institute of Health.

References

1. LeProust EM, Peck BJ, Spirin K et al (2010) Synthesis of high-quality libraries of long (150mer) oligonucleotides by a novel depurination controlled process. Nucleic Acids Res 38:2522–2540

2. Carr PA, Church GM (2009) Genome engineering. Nat Biotechnol 27:1151–1162

3. Czar MJ, Anderson JC, Bader JS et al (2009) Gene synthesis demystified. Trends Biotechnol 27:63–72

4. Xiong A-S, Peng R-H, Zhuang J et al (2008) Chemical gene synthesis: strategies, softwares, error corrections, and applications. FEMS Microbiol Rev 32:522–540

5. Stemmer WP, Crameri A, Ha KD et al (1995) Single-step assembly of a gene and entire plasmid from large numbers of oligodeoxyribonucleotides. Gene 164:49–53

6. Grisedale K, van Daal A (2014) Linear amplification of target prior to PCR for improved low template DNA results. Biotechniques 56:145–147

7. Lee Z-B, Firnhaber C, Clarke J et al (2015) Gene and library synthesis without amplification: polymerase step reaction (PSR). Biotechniques 59:163–166

8. Hostomský Z, Smrt J, Arnold L et al (1987) Solid-phase assembly of cow colostrum trypsin inhibitor gene. Nucleic Acids Res 15:4849–4856

9. Lundqvist M, Edfors F, Sivertsson Å et al (2015) Solid-phase cloning for high-throughput assembly of single and multiple DNA parts. Nucleic Acids Res 43, e49

10. Xiong A-S, Peng R-H, Zhuang J et al (2008) Non-polymerase-cycling-assembly-based chemical gene synthesis: strategies, methods, and progress. Biotechnol Adv 26:121–134

11. Van den Brulle J, Fischer M, Langmann T et al (2008) A novel solid phase technology for high-throughput gene synthesis. Biotechniques 45:340–343

12. Zhou L, Myers AN, Vandersteen JG et al (2004) Closed-tube genotyping with unlabeled oligonucleotide probes and a saturating DNA dye. Clin Chem 50:1328–1335

13. Rydzanicz R, Zhao XS, Johnson PE (2005) Assembly PCR oligo maker: a tool for design-

ing oligodeoxynucleotides for constructing long DNA molecules for RNA production. Nucleic Acids Res 33:W521–W525

14. Rouillard J-M, Lee W, Truan G et al (2004) Gene2Oligo: oligonucleotide design for in vitro gene synthesis. Nucleic Acids Res 32:W176–W180

15. Kibbe WA (2007) OligoCalc: an online oligonucleotide properties calculator. Nucleic Acids Res 35:W43–W46

16. Ma S, Saaem I, Tian J (2012) Error correction in gene synthesis technology. Trends Biotechnol 30:147–154

17. Horton RM, Hunt HD, Ho SN et al (1989) Engineering hybrid genes without the use of restriction enzymes: gene splicing by overlap extension. Gene 77:61–68

18. Ho SN, Hunt HD, Horton RM et al (1989) Site-directed mutagenesis by overlap extension using the polymerase chain reaction. Gene 77:51–59

Chapter 11

Clonetegration Using OSIP Plasmids: One-Step DNA Assembly and Site-Specific Genomic Integration in Bacteria

Lun Cui and Keith E. Shearwin

Abstract

Clonetegration is a method for site-specific insertion of DNA into prokaryotic chromosomes, based on bacteriophage integrases. The method combines DNA cloning/assembly and chromosomal integration into a single step, providing a simple and rapid strategy for inserting DNA sequences into bacterial chromosomes.

Key words Bacteriophage integrase, Genome engineering, Genome editing, Synthetic biology, Clonetegration

1 Introduction

Insertion of DNA sequences into bacterial chromosomes has several advantages over the use of plasmids, in areas such as the study of gene regulation, in metabolic engineering, and particularly in the emerging field of synthetic biology. The advantages of chromosomal integration include a reduction in plasmid copy number variation from cell to cell within a bacterial population, a reduced metabolic burden on the host, and perhaps most significantly eliminating the need for continued antibiotic selection. As progress in synthetic biology demands evermore complex genetic manipulation of bacterial strains [1–3], new rapid and scalable genome editing tools are required. In this chapter we describe such a tool, based on bacteriophage-derived integrases which normally mediate recombination between *attB* sequences in the bacterial chromosome and an *attP* sequence on the phage. When placed on a plasmid, the same *attP* sequences direct the integration of the plasmid into the chromosomal *attB* sequence. Clonetegration, which combines DNA cloning/assembly and chromosomal integration into one single procedure, enables the simple insertion of target DNA sequences into the bacterial chromosome without plasmid propagation and purification [4, 5].

Randall A. Hughes (ed.), *Synthetic DNA: Methods and Protocols*, Methods in Molecular Biology, vol. 1472,
DOI 10.1007/978-1-4939-6343-0_11, © Springer Science+Business Media New York 2017

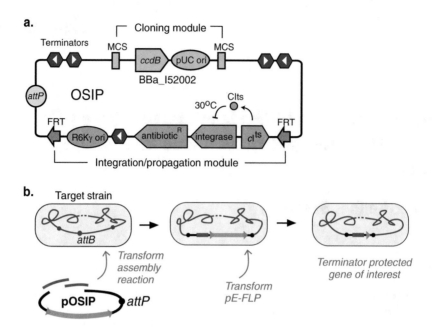

Fig. 1 The clonetegration process. (**a**) The structure of a basic pOSIP plasmid. The CI*ts*-controlled integrase gene allows the plasmid to catalyze its own integration into the bacterial chromosome. (**b**) An aliquot of an assembly reaction, with an OSIP backbone and one or more DNA fragments of interest, is transformed into chemically or electrocompetent cells. The plasmid will integrate via its *attP* site into a specific *attB* site in the chromosome, catalyzed by the corresponding integrase. All unwanted OSIP sequence is removed by simple transformation with a pE-FLP plasmid, leaving only the terminator-protected sequence in the chromosome. Reprinted in modified form with permission from [4]. Copyright (2013) American Chemical Society

Clonetegration utilizes the one-step integration plasmid (OSIP) series of vectors, originally developed by combining and optimizing key features from the well-known CRIM system of Haldiman and Wanner [6]. The OSIP vectors have two functional modules [4] (Fig. 1): the integration/propagation module and the cloning module. The integration/propagation module contains the site-specific recombinase gene, under the control of the lambda CI*ts* repressor, and the corresponding *attP* attachment sequence. It also contains an antibiotic selection marker and the R6Kγ origin of replication. R6Kγ is a conditional replication origin, only functional in a strain carrying the *pir* gene [7], thus allowing propagation of OSIP as a plasmid (if required) in a *pir*⁺ strain, but stable integration of the plasmid into the chromosome of any strain lacking the *pir* gene. The cloning module has a split multiple cloning site (MCS) containing BioBricks element BBa_I52002 [8], a sequence which carries both a mini *pUC* origin to allow high DNA yields of the unmodified plasmid, and a *ccdB* gene, used as a negative selection marker. The *ccdB* gene, which expresses a toxin targeting the essential DNA gyrase [9], helps to minimize background integration.

The modular integration/propagation cassettes can easily be exchanged in the event that different *attB* sites or selection markers are required. The region of the plasmid containing the integration/propagation module is flanked by FRT sites, facilitating its efficient removal via a simple transformation with a FLP plasmid specifically developed for use with the OSIP vectors. Removal of this module thus allows further rounds of OSIP integrations at other *attB* sites, reusing the same selection marker if desired.

Here we describe in detail the procedure for assembling and integrating an OSIP plasmid, followed by removal of the integration/propagation module from the integrant, to leave just the terminator protected sequence of interest in the chromosome (Fig. 1). As an example, here we describe pOSIP-KO (kanamycin selection marker; phage 186 attachment site), into which we assemble a pBla-β-galactosidase cassette.

2   Materials

Prepare all solutions using ultrapure water and analytical grade reagents. Carefully follow all local waste disposal regulations when disposing of waste materials.

1. pOSIP plasmids: The pOSIP plasmids (five possible attachment sites; Table 1) and the pE-FLP plasmid are available from Addgene, either individually (*see* **Note 1**) or as a set (*see* **Note 2**). Glycerol stocks of the strains should be made and stored at –80 °C (*see* **Note 3**).

Table 1

The OSIP series of vectors which carry a kanamycin selection cassette and various integration modules

Name	Integrase/*attP*	Antibiotic	Unique restriction sites in left MCS	Unique restriction sites in right MCS
pOSIP-KO	186 (O)	Kanamycin (K)	EcoRI, Acc65I, KpnI, BamHI	SpeI, PstI, SphI, KasI, NarI, SfoI
pOSIP-KH	HK022 (H)	Kanamycin (K)	EcoRI, Acc65I, KpnI, SacI, BamHI	SpeI, PstI, SphI, XhoI, KasI, NarI, SfoI
pOSIP-KL	lambda (L)	Kanamycin (K)	EcoRI, Acc65I, KpnI, SacI	SpeI, PstI, SphI, XhoI, KasI, NarI, SfoI
pOSIP-KP	Φ 80 (P)	Kanamycin (K)	EcoRI, Acc65I, KpnI, SacI, SacII	PstI, KasI, NarI, SfoI
pOSIP-KT	P21 (T)	Kanamycin (K)	EcoRI, Acc65I, KpnI, SacI, BamHI	SpeI, PstI, XhoI, KasI, NarI, SfoI

The relevant restriction enzymes which can be used to linearize the OSIPs by endonuclease enzyme digestion are also indicated. Note that other OSIP backbones with different selection cassettes are available (*see* **Note 1**)

2. LB medium (for making 1 L): 10 g of tryptone, 5 g of yeast extract, 5 g NaCl, in 1 L H_2O. Adjust to pH 7.2, and autoclave for 15 min at 121 °C on liquid cycle. Store at room temperature.

3. LB-agar: LB containing 1.5% (w/v) agar. For preparing LB-agar plates in Petri dishes (90 mm × 15 mm), LB-agar is melted in a microwave oven and the bottle placed in a water bath set at 48 °C (*see* **Note 4**). When the LB-agar has cooled to the temperature of the water bath, antibiotics and/or X-gal (if screening for β-galactosidase activity) is added from a 1000× stock solution. To pour LB-agar plates, 20 mL of melted LB-agar is poured into each plate on a level surface and the lids replaced quickly to avoid contamination. LB-agar should be allowed to solidify and ideally plates should be dried (overnight at 37 °C) before use to allow excess moisture to evaporate. Plates can be stored at 4 °C for up to a month if kept in sealed bags or boxes.

4. TAE buffer (for making 1 L): Mix 4.84 g of Tris base, 1.14 mL of glacial acetic acid, and 2 mL of 0.5 M EDTA (pH 8.0), and add H_2O to 1 L. Autoclave and store at room temperature (*see* **Note 5**).

5. TAE-agarose gel (for making 100 mL 1% (w/v) TAE-agarose gel): Weigh 1.0 g agarose and resuspend it in 100 mL of 1× TAE buffer. Boil the TAE-agarose mixture until the agarose is completely dissolved. Cool the boiled TAE-agarose mixture to around 55 °C, and then pour into a casting apparatus (including a tray and a comb). Wait until the gel has solidified completely before use (*see* **Note 6**).

6. DNA size markers for agarose gel electrophoresis: We use a 2-log ladder from New England Biolabs (Ipswich, MA), as these markers cover a wide range of DNA sizes from 100 to 10,000 bp.

7. Restriction enzymes, as required by the specific cloning strategy employed. In the example given here, we use EcoRI and PstI from NEB (*see* Table 1).

8. A plasmid miniprep kit, such as the Qiagen Qiaspin Miniprep kit.

9. A DNA gel extraction Kit, such as the Zymoclean Gel DNA Recovery Kit (Zymo Research).

10. A high-fidelity proofreading thermostable DNA polymerase for generating DNA fragments by PCR. We use a KAPA HiFi PCR kit, which includes the correct buffer and the required dNTP mix (Kapa Biosystems).

11. Isothermal assembly master mixture: Commercially prepared Gibson assembly master mix can be used, but we find it more economical to prepare it in-house. The 5× isothermal (ISO) buffer: 25% (w/v) PEG8000, 500 mM Tris–HCl pH 7.5, 50 mM $MgCl_2$, 50 mM DTT, 1 mM each of the four dNTPs (New

England Biolabs (NEB)), and 5 mM NAD (NEB). To prepare 1.2 mL of isothermal assembly master mix, combine the following: 320 μL 5× ISO buffer, 0.64 μL of 10 U/μL T5 exonuclease (Epicentre), 20 μL of 2 U/μL Phusion polymerase (NEB), and 160 μL of 40 U/μL Taq DNA ligase (NEB) and add water to a final volume of 1.2 mL [10]. The master mixture was aliquoted into 15 μL aliquots in 200 μL PCR tubes and stored at −20 °C. This recipe can be used for assembling DNA fragments with overlapping DNA sequences of 20–150 base pairs.

12. Transformation and storage solution (TSS) [11]: LB containing 10% PEG8000 (w/v), 5% DMSO (v/v), and 30 mM MgSO₄. Adjust the pH to 6.5, and sterilize by filtration through a 0.22 μM filter. TSS solution can also be sterilized by autoclaving. Store in aliquots at −20 °C.

13. DNA polymerase for screening potential integrants by colony PCR: We use the KAPA2G Robust kit which contains all the reagents necessary for the PCR reaction (Kapa Biosystems).

3   Methods

3.1   Generating and Assembling DNA Fragments

1. Select an appropriate OSIP vector (*see* **Note 7**). Two criteria must be considered when making this decision. First, the corresponding *attB* integration site in the preferred host strain must not be already occupied, either by a prophage or another integrant. Second, the host strain must not carry the same antibiotic resistance gene as the OSIP vector. Here, the insertion of a pBla-LacZ DNA fragment (containing the constitutive β-lactamase promoter driving expression of the *lacZ* gene) into *E. coli* 186 *attB* site was used as an example (*see* **Note 8**).

2. Grow a 3 mL culture of the host strain carrying pOSIP-KO-I52002 DNA in LB + kanamycin (50 μg/mL) at 30 °C overnight.

3. Isolate pOSIP-KO-I52002 plasmid DNA using a standard miniprep kit, such as the Qiagen Qiaprep Spin miniprep kit (*see* **Note 9**).

4. Digest approximately 500 ng of pOSIP-KO-I52002 with 5 U of EcoRI and 5 U of PstI restriction enzymes in the 1× buffer supplied with the enzymes, in a total volume of 40 μL. The digestion reaction mixture was incubated at 37 °C for 2 h.

5. Inactivate the enzymes by incubating the digestion reaction mixture at 80 °C for 20 min.

6. Check the digestion. Load 10% of the digestion reaction volume on a 1% TAE-agarose gel alongside DNA markers, such as a 2-log ladder. For these gels, DNA can be either pre-stained (e.g., EZ-vision from AMRESCO) or post-stained (e.g., Gel Red from

Biotium). Two bands should be observed on the DNA gel. The larger band should be 5325 bp (the pOSIP-KO backbone), and the smaller band is 1144 bp (the BBa_I52002 band).

7. Gel extraction and purification of the pOSIP-KO backbone band are performed using a commercial kit, such as the Zymoclean kit, designed to allow elution of the purified product into a small volume. The remainder of the digest is loaded on a freshly poured gel. It is convenient to use preparative gel combs which give larger volume wells. This allows the entire sample to be run in one lane, minimizing the volume of gel that needs to be excised. The gel should be post-stained with fresh SYBRsafe stain and the band excised with a sterile scalpel blade. We followed the manufacturer's protocol carefully, eluting the DNA in 10 μL of elution buffer (*see* **Note 10**). The final concentration of eluted backbone should be estimated by running 1 μL on a gel, or preferably by using a Nanodrop spectrophotometer (Thermo-Fisher).

8. The pBla-LacZ fragment was amplified using as a template an existing plasmid containing this cassette (*see* **Note 11**). Primers for this PCR were designed to have 5′ tails of 25–35 bases which overlap with the OSIP backbone adjacent to the restriction site [10], followed by a 25–30 base sequence which anneals to the template. The 3′ of the primer annealing to the template should have a melting temperature (T_m) of between 55 and 65 °C. A proofreading, high-fidelity DNA polymerase should be used in order to minimize the chances of introducing errors.

9. The 20 μL PCR reactions, set up in 200 μL thin-walled PCR tubes, contain 0.4 U KAPA HiFi DNA Polymerase (Kapa Biosystems, Wilmington, MA), 0.6 μL each primer (from 10 μM stock solutions), 0.6 μL of a 10 mM dNTP mix, 4 μL 5× KAPA HiFi buffer, 0.2 μL template plasmid (0.5 ng/μL), and 13.6 μL H_2O. The following program was used for the PCR reaction: initial denaturing for 3 min at 95 °C; 30 cycles of denaturing at 98 °C for 20 s, primer annealing at 55 °C for 20 s, and extension at 72 °C for 4 min; final extension at 72 °C for 10 min; then hold at 12 °C. Extension time for KAPA HiFi DNA polymerase is given as 30 s/kb by the manufacturer.

10. Check PCR products by loading 1 μL of the PCR reaction on a TAE-agarose (1%) gel, along with 2-log ladder DNA size markers. The target band in this instance is a 4590 bp fragment. The amplified DNA fragments can be purified by gel extraction, as described above for the vector backbone. Final concentrations of the eluted fragments should be determined using a Nanodrop spectrophotometer (*see* **Note 12**).

11. Assemble the linearized OSIP backbone and target DNA sequences using isothermal assembly (*see* **Note 13**). Add equimolar amount of pOSIP-KO backbone and pBla-LacZ fragment into

a thawed 15 µL isothermal assembly master mix. In this assembly, 50 ng pOSIP-KO backbone and 45 ng pBla-LacZ fragment were added into the pre-made master mixture. Make the reaction up to a final volume of 20 µL with H_2O. Incubate the isothermal assembly reaction mixture at 50 °C for 1 h (*see* **Note 14**).

3.2 Transformation of the Assembly Product

1. Preparing competent cells: Start a fresh overnight culture (2 mL in LB) of the target strain (*see* **Note 15**) (here MG1655, with a deletion of the lacZYA region [12]) from an isolated colony on a freshly streaked plate. Next day, dilute 1:100 into LB media (for example, 1 mL of overnight culture into 99 mL LB media). Incubate at 37 °C with shaking (at approximately 200 rpm). When the diluted culture has grown to an OD_{600} between 0.4 and 0.6, place the culture on ice for 10 min. Centrifuge the cells at $4000 \times g$ for 10 min at 4 °C to pellet. Discard the supernatant, and gently resuspend the cells in 1/10 volume of ice-cold TSS buffer. It is crucial to keep the cells cold at all times. Aliquot the cells (50 µL) into precooled Eppendorf tubes and use on the same day or freeze at −80 °C for later use (*see* **Note 16**).

2. Gently mix a 5 µL aliquot of the isothermal assembly reaction (Subheading 3.1, **step 11**) with a 50 µL aliquot of TSS chemically competent cells in a precooled 1.5 mL Eppendorf tube on ice. Incubate on ice for 20–30 min. In a modification to the original protocol [11], the cells are heat shocked by placing the tubes at 42 °C in a heating block for 45 s. One milliliter of LB media is added immediately and the cells incubated at 37 °C for 1 h with shaking (150 rpm). Incubation at 37 °C inactivates the CI*ts* repressor, and allows expression of the integrase from the OSIP plasmid. Although lambda CI*ts* repressor is not completely inactivated at 37 °C, incubation at higher temperatures during the recovery phase does not produce a significant improvement in integration efficiency.

3. Spread 200 µL of the transformation mix on an LB-agar plus kanamycin (20 µg/mL) plate. For larger plasmid sizes where integration efficiency may be lower, more of the transformation mix can be plated out. Incubate the plate at 30 °C overnight. Incubation at this lower temperature ensures that repression of integrase expression is re-established (*see* **Note 17**).

3.3 Screening for Correct Integration

1. Next day, record the number of colonies observed. Restreak isolated single colonies from the overnight plate onto a fresh LB-agar kanamycin (20 µg/mL) plate. Incubate the restreaked plate at 30 °C overnight. Restreaking is necessary to ensure that a single clone is isolated, and also to ensure that any transformed but unintegrated OSIP plasmid (which is unable to replicate extra-chromosomally) has been lost as a result of several cell divisions (*see* **Note 18**).

2. Set up colony PCR reactions to screen for correct integrants. Each 10 μL PCR colony reaction contained the following: 0.04 μL of 5 U/μL KAPA2G Robust DNA Polymerase (Kapa Biosystems), 0.8 μL of a stock solution containing the fours primers P1 to P4 (100 ng/μL of each primer) (Fig. 2, Table 2), 0.2 μL dNTPs (10 mM), 2 μL of 5× KAPA 2G buffer B (Kapa Biosystems), and 6.96 μL H$_2$O (*see* **Note 19**). If using a master mix, aliquot 10 μL per tube, on ice.

3. Use sterile wire/yellow pipette tip/toothpick to pick a small portion of an isolated colony from the restreaked plate, ensuring that the colony chosen is clearly identified by a number/name written on the underside of the plate (*see* **Note 20**). Swirl the colony into the correspondingly labeled tube of PCR master mix. Kapa2G Robust DNA polymerase is designed specifically for colony PCRs; however taking too much colony can inhibit the reaction.

4. Transfer reactions into a thermocycler and start the reactions using the following: initial denaturing for 3 min at 95 °C; 30 cycles of denaturing at 95 °C for 20 s, primer annealing at

a. *Plasmid*

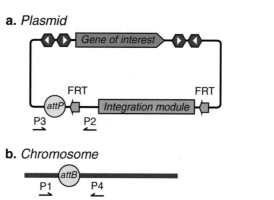

b. *Chromosome*

c. *Single integrant*

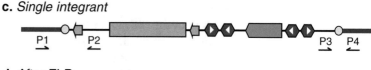

d. *After FLP*

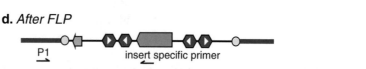

Fig. 2 Screening for integration by PCR. The figure shows the positions of primers used to verify single-copy chromosomal integration. Primer positions are indicated in (**a**) plasmid, (**b**) chromosome, (**c**) a single integrant, and (**d**) a single integrant following successful FLP-mediated excision of the sequence between the FRT sites. Expected sizes for the PCR products for each *attB* site are given in Table 3. Reprinted in modified form with permission from [4]. Copyright (2013) American Chemical Society

Table 2

PCR primer sequences used for screening chromosomal integrations

attB site	Primer P1	Primer P2	Primer P3	Primer P4
186 (O) (primary)	CTCATTCGAAACCACC CACCG	ACTTAACGGCTGACATGG	ACGAGTATCGAGATGGCA	GATCATCATGTTTATTGCGTGG
HK022 (H)	GGAATCAATGCCTGAGTG	ACTTAACGGCTGACATGG	ACGAGTATCGAGATGGCA	GGCATCAACAGCACATTC
Lambda (L)	GGCATCACGGCAATATAC	ACTTAACGGCTGACATGG	GGGAATTAATTCTTGA AGACG	TCTGGTCTGGTAGCAATG
Φ80 (P)	GATTTGAGCGAGCAA CTGTACC	GTTCGCAGAGTGT TATGGTT	AAAGAAACAGAGAAGG GCAC	TGGCCTTAACAAAGACATCA
P21 (T)	ATCGCCTGTATGAACCTG	ACTTAACGGCTGACATGG	GGGAATTAATTCT TGAAGACG	TAGAACTACCACCTGACC
186 (O) (secondary)	TCCGGAATGCCTGCATTG	ACTTAACGGCTGACATGG	ACGAGTATCGAGATGGCA	CCCTGGAGCCAAAATATCC

Table 3

Expected product sizes (in base pairs) when screening for chromosomal integration events by PCR

Integration site	No integration P1 and P4 (attB)	Single integration P1 and P2	Single integration P3 and P4	Additional band in tandem integrants P2 and P3
186 (O) (primary site)	241	389	328	476
HK022(H)	740	343	824	427
Lambda (L)	741	631	1156	1046
Φ80 (P)	569	303	499	233
P21 (T)	506	622	1110	1226
186 (O) (secondary site)	601	648	429	476

For a correct integration event, two PCR products (P1/P2 and P3/P4) will be observed

55 °C for 20 s, and extension at 72 °C for 2 min; final extension at 72 °C for 10 min; then hold at 12 °C.

5. Load 5 µL of each PCR reaction (with an appropriate loading dye added) along with a lane of DNA size markers such as 2-log ladder (NEB) onto a TAE-agarose (2%) gel. Run the gel at 120 V until the dyes in the loading buffer are appropriately separated.

6. Compare the size of the PCR products with Table 3. Two bands (*attL* and *attR*) of the correct size indicate a single integration event. If only one band is observed (the *attB* band), there is no integration. If three bands are observed, there are two tandem copies in this *att* site. Typically, we screen five colonies from a given clonetegration and the majority are correct integrants. Tandem copies are rare.

7. Store the correct integrants as glycerol stocks in a −80 °C freezer.

3.4 Removing the OSIP Backbone Using pE-FLP

1. Grow a 3 mL overnight culture (LB plus ampicillin 100 µg/mL) **at 30 °C** of the strain carrying the pE-FLP plasmid (*see* Note 21).

2. Next day, prepare a miniprep of the pE-FLP plasmid using the Qiagen Qiaspin Miniprep kit. No modifications to the standard protocol are required. Measure the concentration of the pE-FLP plasmid prep using a Nanodrop spectrophotometer, or estimate the concentration by running a 5 µL aliquot on a 1% TAE gel alongside a known amount of DNA size marker.

3. Grow a 3 mL overnight culture (30 °C; LB+kanamycin 20 µg/mL) each of the integrant strains which are to have the OSIP backbone removed.

4. Make the integrant strains chemically competent using the TSS method as described in Subheading 3.2 above. Transform each strain with 20 ng of the pE-FLP plasmid. Allow the transformed cells to recover for at least 30 min at 30 °C.

5. Spread the transformed cells on LB agar plates containing ampicillin (100 µg/mL). Incubate the plate at 30 °C overnight. The FLP-mediated excision occurs during growth of the colony overnight.

6. To check for successful excision of the integration/selection module, restreak an isolated single colony onto three different plates in the following order: LB plus kanamycin (20 µg/mL) plate, LB plus ampicillin (100 µg/mL) plate, and LB (no antibiotic) plate. Incubate these three plates at 42 °C for 2 h, and then move to a 37 °C incubator for overnight growth. Several (4 or 8) colonies can be restreaked onto each individual plate.

7. Next day, check the cell growth on the three different plates. If the pOSIP-KO backbone was successfully removed, cells will not grow on the plates containing kanamycin, but will grow on the no-antibiotic LB plate. Lack of growth on the LB plus ampicillin plate indicates that the Amp-resistant pE-FLP plasmid has been successfully lost, as it cannot replicate at 37 °C. We find that successful removal of the OSIP backbone approaches 100 % when using the pE-FLP plasmid (*see* **Note 22**).

8. Make an overnight culture of the successfully "flipped" strains. Use a sterile toothpick to pick isolated colonies from the LB plate. Dip the toothpick into 3 mL LB and swirl gently to inoculate the culture. Ensure the use of sterile technique at this stage, as the strains no longer carry any antibiotic resistance marker. Incubate the tube in 37 °C overnight (*see* **Note 23**).

9. Mix 500 µL of 80 % glycerol with 500 µL of overnight culture in a glycerol storage tube, mix by inversion, and store at −80 °C.

4 Notes

1. Plasmids are available from Addgene at https://www.add-gene.org/posip/#kit-contents. There are six OSIP plasmids available with a kanamycin marker (Table 1), two with a chloramphenicol marker and two with tetracycline marker. Plasmid maps and full sequence are available on the Addgene website. Other combinations of attachment site and selection marker can easily be made by DNA assembly if required. Ampicillin selection is not used on the OSIP plasmids, as this marker is reserved for use with the FLP plasmid.

2. Note that pOSIP-phiC31, included as part of the OSIP collection from Addgene, integrates into the phiC31 *attB* site, which is not found in *E. coli*. Thus, the pOSIP-phiC31 plasmid should not be used for routine integrations, unless the phiC31 *att* site has artificially been engineered into the strain of interest.

3. To prepare glycerol stocks for long-term storage, strains carrying the OSIP plasmids or the pE-FLP plasmid should be cultured overnight in LB, with appropriate antibiotic selection at *30 °C*. Glycerol stocks are prepared by adding equal volumes of overnight culture, and sterile 80% (v/v) glycerol to a sterile screw capped tube, mixing well by inversion, and storing at –80 °C.

4. To melt solid LB-agar in the microwave, always ensure that the bottle lid is loose and use short periods of heating, followed by gentle swirling of the bottle. Always wear personal protective equipment, including eye protection and use sturdy heat-resistant gloves.

5. If many gels are to be run, it is often convenient to make a 5× or 10× stock solution of TAE buffer, and dilute to 1× prior to use.

6. The concentration of agarose should be adjusted depending on the size of the fragments of interest. For fragments below 500 bp, a 2% (w/v) agarose gel should be used. Use a good-quality agarose, particularly if the gel will be used for a gel extraction procedure to isolate DNA for assembly.

7. The unmodified OSIP plasmids, containing the BBa_I5200 Biobrick element (pUC origin and *ccdB* gene), are supplied, and should be propagated in, a strain such as DB3.1 (Life Technologies) which carries a mutation enabling growth in the presence of the gyrase toxin *ccdB* [9]. Removal of the BBa_ I5200 element during cloning gives a plasmid containing just the R6Kγ origin, which can only replicate in a *pir+* strain. If multicopy propagation of the modified OSIP plasmids is required, they can be transformed into a *pir+* strain such as TransformMax EC100D *pir+* for replication at approximately 15 copies per cell or TransforMax EC100D *pir*-116, for replication at ~250 copies per cell (Epicentre, Madison, WI). To avoid the risk of selecting for mutations, propagation at high copy number should be avoided if there is a possibility that the gene product inserted into the MCS of the OSIP plasmid might be toxic to the host cell. Note that it is important to grow cultures carrying the OSIP plasmids at *30 °C*, in order to maintain repression of integrase expression by the temperature-sensitive lambda repressor.

8. *E. coli* contains two phage 186 *attB* sequences, one in the *tRNA IleY* gene and a second in the *tRNA IleX* gene [4, 13]. These can easily be distinguished by PCR, using primers given in Table 2.

9. No modifications to the standard miniprep procedure are required. The unmodified pOSIP-KO-I52002 plasmid replicates using the pUC origin, and so a 3 mL overnight culture, will yield ample DNA for subsequent steps. The DNA concentration (and yield) can be estimated by running a 5 μL aliquot of the miniprep on a 1% agarose gel, or by use of a small-volume spectrophotometer, such as one of the Nanodrop series of spectrophotometers (Thermo Scientific).

10. No modifications to the standard gel extraction and elution protocol were employed; however exposure of the DNA to UV light should be minimized or preferably eliminated during band excision. We routinely use an LED-based light box (e.g., Safe Imager 2.0, Life Technologies) with a narrow emission peak centered at 470 nm wavelength, which is compatible with SYBR Safe nucleic acid stain.

11. Other methods can also be used to generate the DNA fragments for assembly. For example, the vector backbone can be prepared by amplifying it using PCR. Similarly, the fragments to be inserted into the OSIP vector can also be generated by other methods, such as conventional restriction digest (if appropriate sites are available) and DNA or gene synthesis. Linear double-stranded DNA fragments (such as g-blocks from IDT) produced by DNA synthesis can be cost-effective ways of producing the insert fragments, particularly if no natural source of the desired sequence is available for use as a template in a PCR. The quantity of these types of DNA fragments provided by the vendors is relatively low (a few hundred nanograms), which is sufficient for perhaps 6–8 assembly reactions. If many assembly reactions are required using the same DNA fragment, then gene synthesis where the requested DNA sequence is provided cloned into a vector should be considered.

12. The PCR fragments can also be purified by a spin column cleanup procedure, such as the Zymo DNA Clean and Concentrate kit. If the PCR reactions produce clean, strong bands of the correct size, unpurified PCR reaction can be used directly in the subsequent assembly reaction.

13. Here, the Gibson isothermal assembly method [10] was used to generate the desired OSIP vector. The advantage of Gibson assembly is that clone design is not limited by the availability of a limited set of restriction sites. The isothermal assembly method is also highly efficient for multiple fragment assembly. We have successfully assembled up to seven individual fragments. However, any other DNA assembly method, including conventional restriction/ligation, in-fusion cloning [14], USER cloning [15], or ligase cycling reaction [16] can be used to generate the final OSIP plasmid to be integrated.

14. If all DNA fragments, including the plasmid backbone, have been generated by PCR, the completed assembly reaction can be treated with DpnI restriction enzyme. DpnI will digest methylated DNA, such as plasmid DNA, but will not digest unmethylated DNA, such as PCR products. Thus DpnI treatment (addition of 0.5 μL of DpnI directly to the completed assembly reaction, followed by incubation for 30 min at 37 °C) will destroy any methylated plasmid molecules, used as templates in the PCR reactions which may have carried through the gel extraction process. If they carry the same antibiotic resistance marker as the assembled product, any supercoiled template molecules will transform efficiently and can contribute to a high count of background colonies following transformation. It is useful to perform a control assembly reaction, where all the fragments are added to H_2O, rather than isothermal assembly mix. Transformation of this reaction will only give colonies in the event that parental template DNA has carried through.

15. Here, we used *E. coli* K12 MG1655 strain as an example [12]. Essentially any strain of *E. coli* can be used subject to the constraints outlined in Subheading 3.1. In the original publication [4], we also showed successful integration of DNA sequences into *Salmonella typhimurium* using OSIP.

16. Other standard methods of making chemically competent cells, such as the calcium chloride method [17], can also be used. We prefer the TSS method because the cells are prepared simply by resuspending them directly in TSS solution; they are ready for immediate use, and can be stored at –80 °C in TSS solution for later use. In-house electrocompetent cells can be prepared by standard methods [18], and give higher efficiency of integration for larger constructs. Commercially available chemically competent cells represent a useful alternative, as the volume of the transformation reaction can be scaled down to save on costs, and transformation efficiencies are considerably higher than can be obtained in-house. Finally, commercial electrocompetent cells can be used, and will give the highest efficiency of transformation, but are relatively expensive.

17. Because integrants are present at single copy in the bacterial chromosome, the antibiotic concentrations used for selection should be lower than normally used for selecting multicopy plasmids. We suggest the following antibiotic concentrations for selecting single-copy integrants: kanamycin (20 μg/mL), chloramphenicol (20 μg/mL), and tetracycline (10 μg/mL).

18. If no colonies (integrants) are observed, the transformation can be repeated with electrocompetent cells. If so, the assembly mix should first be desalted by passage through a DNA cleanup spin column, such as a Zymo Clean and Concentrate

kit (Zymo Research). If again no colonies are observed, an aliquot of the assembly mix should be transformed (at 30 °C) into a *pir⁺* strain, such as TransformMax EC100D *pir⁺* (Epicentre) in which OSIP cannot integrate, but can replicate as a plasmid. In this way the assembled plasmid can be checked by PCR and/or sequencing prior to integration. If correct, a miniprep can be performed and the OSIP plasmid DNA transformed and integrated into the desired strain, a process which gives a higher efficiency of integration. This approach, while slower, has the advantage that a stock of the correct plasmid is available (as a DNA miniprep or as a frozen glycerol stock of the *pir⁺* strain) for later use.

19. When screening *n* colonies across multiple clonetegrations, it is convenient to prepare a PCR master mix, preparing a volume of master mix sufficient for $n+1$ reactions. Note that in the case of 186, there are two *attB* sites in the *E. coli* chromosome. If a correct single integrant is found at the primary 186 *attB* site, the secondary site should then be screened, using the primers shown in Table 2. In the integrant screening step, PCR can also be used to verify the presence of the inserted fragment within the MCS. This PCR product can then be used as a template to set up a sequencing reaction to confirm that no mutations have been introduced.

20. To simultaneously prepare cultures for each of the colonies to be screened, one can dip the wire/pipette tip/toothpick into 3 mL LB (with 20 μg/mL kanamycin) in 10 mL culture tube, and stir gently three times to resuspend the cells. Dip the same wire/pipette tip/toothpick into the 10 μL PCR reactions.

21. The pE-FLP plasmid carries the yeast FLP recombinase gene under the control of the constitutive pE promoter from phage P2. The plasmid also has a temperature-sensitive origin of replication and is cured simply by growing the strain at 37 °C. This plasmid is supplied (and should be propagated) in a strain which expresses the P2 C repressor, in order to keep the pE promoter repressed. A strain which is lysogenic for the P2 phage is suitable. *It is also critical that the host strain carrying the pE-FLP plasmid is propagated at 30 °C.* At higher temperatures, replication of the plasmid will cease, and it will be lost by dilution as the cells divide.

22. The heat-inducible pCP20 plasmid [19] has been used extensively for FLP-mediated removal of sequences located between FRT sites. However, we found that pCP20 did not work efficiently with the OSIP plasmids. We speculate that this might be due to interference between the CIts-controlled modules which are present on both the OSIP and pCP20 plasmids. For this reason we developed the pE-FLP plasmid, which constitu-

tively expresses FLP, in the absence of the phage P2 C repressor. To confirm correct removal of the OSIP backbone, the final clones can be screened by colony PCR, using the P1 primer (Table 2) and a primer specific for the sequence inserted in the MCS (Fig. 2). In the specific example given here, we used a primer within the lacZ gene (primer FLIP_F: ATCTGGTGCTGGGTCTGGTG).

23. Removal of the integration and selection module sequences between two FRT sites leaves a single FRT scar sequence. If planning to clonetegrate and then flip out several OSIP plasmids, consideration should be given to using *attB* sites widely separated in the chromosome [4]. This will reduce the chances of unwanted recombination events between the remaining FRT scar sites.

Acknowledgements

This work was supported by the Pasteur-Roux Fellowship (L.C.) and Australian Research Council grants DP110100824 and DP110101470 and HFSP grant RGP051 (K.E.S.).

References

1. Bonnet J, Subsoontorn P, Endy D (2012) Rewritable digital data storage in live cells via engineered control of recombination directionality. Proc Natl Acad Sci U S A 109(23):8884–8889. doi:10.1073/pnas.1202344109

2. Nielsen AA, Segall-Shapiro TH, Voigt CA (2013) Advances in genetic circuit design: novel biochemistries, deep part mining, and precision gene expression. Curr Opin Chem Biol 17(6):878–892. doi:10.1016/j.cbpa.2013.10.003

3. Stanton BC, Nielsen AA, Tamsir A et al (2014) Genomic mining of prokaryotic repressors for orthogonal logic gates. Nat Chem Biol 10(2):99–105. doi:10.1038/nchembio.1411

4. St-Pierre F, Cui L, Priest DG et al (2013) One-step cloning and chromosomal integration of DNA. ACS Synth Biol 2(9):537–541. doi:10.1021/sb400021j

5. Cui L, St-Pierre F, Shearwin K (2013) Repurposing site-specific recombinases for synthetic biology. Future Microbiol 8(11):1361–1364. doi:10.2217/fmb.13.119

6. Haldimann A, Wanner BL (2001) Conditional-replication, integration, excision, and retrieval plasmid-host systems for gene structure-function studies of bacteria. J Bacteriol 183(21):6384–6393

7. Filutowicz M, McEachern MJ, Helinski DR (1986) Positive and negative roles of an initiator protein at an origin of replication. Proc Natl Acad Sci U S A 83(24):9645–9649

8. Shetty RP, Endy D, Knight TF Jr (2008) Engineering BioBrick vectors from BioBrick parts. J Biol Eng 2:5. doi:10.1186/1754-1611-2-5

9. Bernard P, Couturier M (1992) Cell killing by the F plasmid CcdB protein involves poisoning of DNA-topoisomerase II complexes. J Mol Biol 226(3):735–745

10. Gibson DG, Young L, Chuang RY et al (2009) Enzymatic assembly of DNA molecules up to several hundred kilobases. Nat Methods 6(5):343–345. doi:10.1038/nmeth.1318

11. Chung CT, Niemela SL, Miller RH (1989) One-step preparation of competent Escherichia coli: transformation and storage of bacterial cells in the same solution. Proc Natl Acad Sci U S A 86(7):2172–2175

12. Priest DG, Cui L, Kumar S et al (2014) Quantitation of the DNA tethering effect in long-range DNA looping in vivo and in vitro using the Lac and lambda repressors. Proc Natl

Acad Sci U S A 111(1):349–354. doi:10.1073/pnas.1317817111

13. Reed MR, Shearwin KE, Pell LM et al (1997) The dual role of Apl in prophage induction of coliphage 186. Mol Microbiol 23(4):669–681

14. Irwin CR, Farmer A, Willer DO et al (2012) In-fusion(R) cloning with vaccinia virus DNA polymerase. Methods Mol Biol 890:23–35. doi:10.1007/978-1-61779-876-4_2

15. Genee HJ, Bonde MT, Bagger FO et al (2015) Software-supported USER cloning strategies for site-directed mutagenesis and DNA assembly. ACS Synth Biol 4(3):342–349. doi:10.1021/sb500194z

16. de Kok S, Stanton LH, Slaby T et al (2014) Rapid and reliable DNA assembly via ligase cycling reaction. ACS Synth Biol 3(2):97–106. doi:10.1021/sb4001992

17. Dagert M, Ehrlich SD (1979) Prolonged incubation in calcium chloride improves the competence of Escherichia coli cells. Gene 6(1):23–28

18. Gonzales MF, Brooks T, Pukatzki SU et al (2013) Rapid protocol for preparation of electrocompetent Escherichia coli and Vibrio cholerae. J Vis Exp 80:PMID:24146001. doi:10.3791/50684

19. Cherepanov PP, Wackernagel W (1995) Gene disruption in Escherichia coli: TcR and KmR cassettes with the option of Flp-catalyzed excision of the antibiotic-resistance determinant. Gene 158(1):9–14

Chapter 12

Generation of DNA Constructs Using the Golden GATEway Cloning Method

Stephan Kirchmaier, Katharina Lust, and Jochen Wittbrodt

Abstract

One of the most frequently executed tasks for molecular biologists is the design and generation of complex DNA constructs. Recently, we established the Golden GATEway cloning kit for the fast and efficient generation of transgenesis vectors. This cloning kit allows the modular assembly of DNA fragments in a defined order. The modularity reflects how complex transgenesis constructs are set up. For example, genome modification tools such as the Cre-Lox system utilize small recombination elements that are combined with larger open reading frames and noncoding regulatory DNA. Another example is that proteinogenic genes can be extended with different localisation tags or fluorescent markers. The Golden GATEway cloning kit allows focusing on the design of a transgenesis construct without having to compromise it by so far available cloning strategies. Here, we provide a step-by-step introduction on how to use the Golden GATEway cloning kit.

Key words PCR, DNA assembly, Vector construction, Plasmid, Transgenesis, Golden GATEway, Cloning

1 Introduction

The Golden GATEway cloning kit [1] combines two widely used cloning techniques, namely Golden Gate cloning [2] and Multisite Gateway cloning (Fig. 1). Golden Gate cloning relies on the activity of type II restriction enzymes, which cut outside of their non-palindromic recognition sequence. Thereby, a 4 bp overhang is created that can be freely chosen. For the Golden Gate assembly, several Golden Gate entry vectors are combined with a Golden Gate destination vector. The enzyme cuts all vectors, thereby releasing either a DNA fragment from the assembly or the vector backbone. Simultaneously, matching overhangs can be ligated using a standard T4 ligase. This enriches properly ligated DNA constructs since these cannot be cut again by the restriction enzyme. In the Golden GATEway cloning kit, we use the enzyme BsaI for the Golden Gate

---

Stephan Kirchmaier and Katharina Lust contributed equally with all other contributors.

Randall A. Hughes (ed.), *Synthetic DNA: Methods and Protocols*, Methods in Molecular Biology, vol. 1472,
DOI 10.1007/978-1-4939-6343-0_12, © Springer Science+Business Media New York 2017

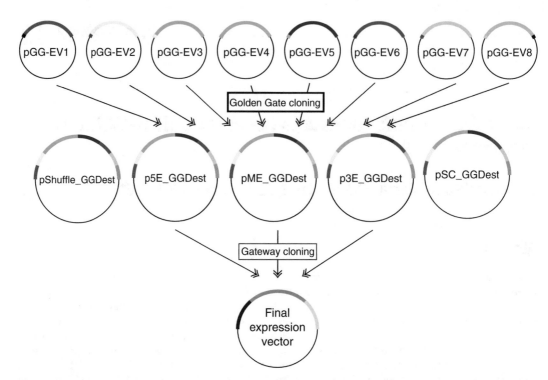

Fig. 1 The principle of Golden GATEway cloning is depicted. Up to eight different DNA fragments in entry vectors are assembled using the Golden Gate cloning method into diverse destination vectors. The pShuffle vector has flanking XcmI sites that allow shuffling the assembly back to any entry vector using standard XcmI restriction and ligation cloning. The pSC destination vector contains few restriction sites enabling further restriction ligation cloning with the Golden Gate assembly. Additionally, the assembly can be prepared in entry vectors for the Multisite Gateway cloning technology at either position. This allows integrating the new assemblies to the already vast resources available for Multisite Gateway cloning to generate the final transgene constructs (Figure adapted from [1])

reaction. A total of eight DNA fragments can be assembled into specific destination vectors. Subsequently, the Golden Gate assembly can be integrated in the widely used Multisite Gateway™ cloning system from Life Technologies. Here, three fragments can be assembled in a defined order using an in vitro recombination system. The major advantage of using Multisite Gateway™ cloning is that vast resources are already available in several vector collections for different species [3–5]. Here, we describe in detail the protocols to generate entry vectors, to assemble the inserts via Golden Gate cloning, and to generate final expression constructs via Multisite Gateway cloning.

2 Materials

2.1 Enzymes

1. FastDigest Eco31I (BsaI) (Thermo Scientific/Life Technologies).

2. FastDigest BamHI (Thermo Scientific/Life Technologies).

3. FastDigest KpnI (Thermo Scientific/Life Technologies).

4. XcmI (New England Biolabs).

5. Taq Polymerase (Roboklon).

6. T4 Polynucleotide Kinase (New England Biolabs).

7. FastAP Alkaline Phosphatase (Thermo Scientific/Life Technologies).

2.2 Chemicals

1. Isopropanol.

2. Ethanol.

3. IPTG: 238.3 mg IPTG in 10 ml H_2O, sterile filtrate, aliquot, and store at –20 °C.

4. X-Gal: 20 mg/ml X-Gal in DMSO, aliquot in dark tubes and store at –20 °C.

5. Ampicillin: 100 mg/ml in 50 % Ethanol.

2.3 Buffers and Media

1. P1 buffer: 50 mM Tris–HCl pH 8.0, 10 mM EDTA pH 8.0, 100 μg/ml RNaseA
   Sterile filter and store at 4 °C.

2. P2 buffer: 0.2 N NaOH, 1 % SDS, sterile filter and store at RT.

3. P3 buffer: 3 M Potassium acetate pH 5.5, adjust pH with glacial acetic acid and store at 4 °C.

4. 10× Oligo annealing buffer: 100 mM Tris–HCl pH 8, 10 mM EDTA pH 8, 1 M NaCl.

5. 10 mM ATP: Dilute the 100 mM ATP stock in water. Aliquot 1 μl for single Golden Gate reactions in PCR tubes and store at –20 °C.

6. 2 mM dATP: Dilute 100 mM dATP stock in 5 mM Tris pH 7.5, prepare small aliquots and store at –20 °C.

7. Lysogeny broth (LB) medium: 10 g/l Bacto-tryptone, 5 g/l yeast extract, 10 g/l sodium chloride.

8. Terrific broth (TB) medium: 12 g/l Bacto-tryptone, 24 g/l yeast extract, 0.4 % glycerin, 2.13 g/l potassium dihydrogen phosphate, 12.54 g/l potassium hydrogen phosphate.

9. LB bacterial agar plates: 10 g/l Bacto-tryptone, 5 g/l yeast extract, 10 g/l sodium chloride, 15 g/l agarose.

2.4 Equipment and Kits

1. Eppendorf tubes.

2. Tabletop centrifuge.

3. Pipettes.

4. Heat block or water bath.

5. Nanodrop (Thermo Scientific).

6. QIAquick PCR Purification Kit (Qiagen).

7. Gateway® LR Clonase® II Plus Enzyme mix (Life Technologies).

3   Methods

3.1   Cloning into Entry Vectors

The first step is to fill the entry vectors with the DNA fragments of choice in order to obtain a library of reusable entry vectors. For that, we included a multiple cloning site with BamHI and KpnI as well as XcmI restriction sites (Fig. 2). These sites flank a LacZ selection gene, enabling blue-white selection of the transformants. The system enables in-frame fusion of the DNA fragments in a prespecified open reading frame. This open reading frame is defined by the 6 bp cutters BamHI and KpnI. If a DNA fragment is in-frame with the BamHI and KpnI sites, then it is in-frame with the entire assembly. The inserts can be cloned into the BamHI and KpnI sites via standard restriction digest of PCR products or vectors. Additionally, these sites can be used to clone annealed oligonucleotides. In some cases, the BamHI and KpnI sites are not usable, if for example the same sites are contained in the insert. Therefore, we included the

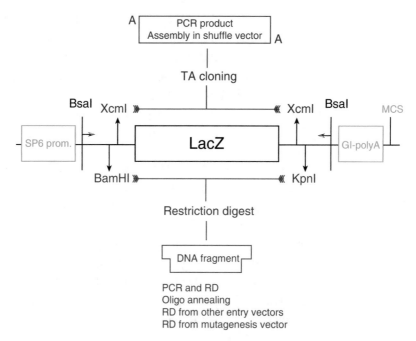

Fig. 2 The different ways to clone into entry vectors are depicted. Importantly, a LacZ gene is included to enable blue-white screening of the colonies. XcmI restriction sites flank the LacZ reporter gene. These leave single T overhangs that allow cloning of PCR products using TA cloning. Furthermore, BamHI and KpnI sites are available for cloning. Importantly, the BamHI and KpnI sites define the final open reading frame in the assembly, thus enabling in-frame assembly. BsaI sites that are used for the Golden Gate assembly then flank this multiple cloning site. Each entry vector contains upstream an Sp6 promoter as well as downstream a rabbit globin intron and SV40 poly A signal (GI-polyA) [6] to generate mRNA from the entry vector inserts (Figure adapted from [1])

option to use TA cloning via an XcmI restriction site. XcmI is a 15 bp cutter that leaves a single-base overhang. PCR products that are generated with a Taq polymerase contain a flanking A overhang that efficiently ligates to the single T overhang established by the XcmI cut. It is designed in such a way that no additional bases need to be added to stay in-frame (*see* **Note 1**).

3.1.1 Cloning into Entry Vectors via BamHI and KpnI

1. The insert is most often not available with the proper BamHI and KpnI flanks. Thus, we routinely use a standard PCR protocol with primers that contain the BamHI and KpnI sites as 5′ attachments (Fig. 3a). For BamHI, any other enzyme with compatible ends such as BglII can be used.

2. Digest 2 µg of the respective entry vector and the entire insert (the DNA fragment for the assembly) with BamHI and KpnI for 1 h at 37 °C.

3. Run the digested vector over a 1% agarose gel. Adapt the percentage of the agarose gel for the insert according to its size.

4. Cut and gel-purify the linearized band of the vector at 4000 bp (*see* **Note 2**).

5. Set up a ligation reaction using 20 ng of the digested vector and three times the molarity of the vector of the insert (*see* **Note 3**).

6. Incubate the ligation for 1 h at RT.

7. Add 1–3 µl of the ligation reaction into 50 µl chemical competent cells that were thawed on ice (*see* **Note 4**).

8. Heat shock the cells for 30 s at 42 °C without shaking in a thermomixer or water bath.

9. Place the tubes on ice for at least 2 min.

10. Add 200 µl pre-warmed TB medium.

11. Shake horizontally at 37 °C for 1 h in a shaking incubator.

12. Plate at least half of the transformed cells on a pre-warmed ampicillin-selective plate and incubate overnight at 37 °C. For the blue-white selection, add 40 µl X-Gal to the plates (*see* **Note 5**).

13. Pick 2–4 white colonies in 2.5 ml LB medium with ampicillin and let them grow for 5–7 h in a shaking incubator at 37 °C (180 rpm).

14. Prepare the miniprep.

    (a) Spin down 2 ml of the bacterial culture (should be cloudy) in a 2 ml Eppendorf tube at $10,000 \times g$ for 3 min. A bacterial pellet will form.

    (b) Discard the supernatant and dissolve the pellet in 250 µl P1 buffer by vortexing or pipetting with a 1 ml pipette tip. Make sure that no cell clumps remain.

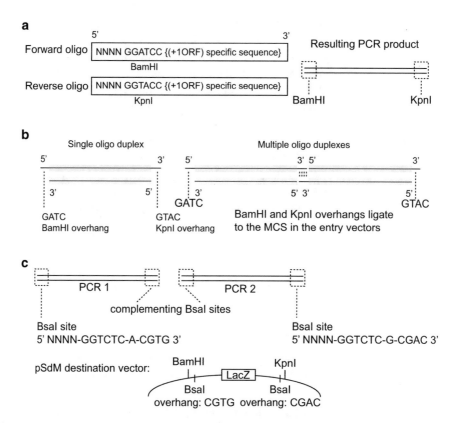

Fig. 3 The oligonucleotide design is illustrated. (**a**) DNA fragments are amplified via a PCR reaction. The oligos contain BamHI as well as KpnI restriction sites at the 5′ end. The flanking 4 bp (NNNN) are important so that the restriction enzymes can cut faithfully at DNA ends. The resulting PCR product is flanked by BamHI and KpnI sites that can be used to insert the DNA fragment into the entry vector. (**b**) Single- as well as multiple-oligo duplexes can be annealed and cloned into the BamHI and KpnI sites. The design of the oligos is depicted. The shaded part of the bottom oligo is reverse complement to the shaded part of the top oligo. Note the established overhangs. Multiple-oligo duplexes can also be cloned when including complementary overhangs between them. (**c**) A site-directed mutagenesis vector allows generating BamHI- and KpnI-flanked DNA fragments by assembling several PCR products with Golden Gate cloning. Here, the BsaI site has to be attached to the oligo so that specific overhangs are created. Note that the ligation to the pSdM vectors utilizes specific overhangs (CGTG and CGAC, respectively). After the Golden Gate reaction, the BamHI and KpnI sites are used to release the assembled fragment and paste it into any entry vector

(c) Add 250 μl P2 buffer and mix by inverting the tube 5–10 times. The solution will be viscous. Do not vortex at this stage to inhibit contamination from the bacterial genomic DNA.

(d) Add 250 μl P3 buffer. A white precipitate will form.

(e) Centrifuge the tubes at maximum speed for 8 min.

(f) Transfer the liquid phase (700 μl) to a 1.5 ml tube with a 1 ml pipette tip. The precipitate will attach to the pipette tip; thus do not touch the wall of the tube with the tip.

(g) Add 650 μl isopropanol and mix by vortexing.

(h) Centrifuge at maximum speed for 20 min. A small DNA pellet will form.

(i) Remove the supernatant and add 1 ml 70% ethanol.

(j) Centrifuge at maximum speed for 10 min.

(k) Remove the supernatant and let the pellet dry.

(l) Resuspend the pellet in 50 μl H2O.

(m) For a test restriction digest use 2.5 μl of the miniprep in a 10 μl reaction. Load the complete reaction on an agarose gel for analysis of the restriction pattern.

3.1.2 Cloning into Entry Vectors via TA Cloning

1. PCR amplify your insert of interest using a Taq polymerase to create A overhangs. Do not add bases to remain in-frame. The A overhang that is attached via the Taq polymerase is taken into account.

2. Alternatively, prepare the PCR reaction with a proofreading polymerase such as Q5 (NEB). Then, the A overhang can be attached with the following steps:

   (a) Set up the PCR reaction and then purify it with a PCR. Elute the PCR product with 30 μl H_2O. Then prepare the A-tailing reaction:

   7.25 μl Purified PCR reaction.

   1 μl 10× Polymerase buffer (supplemented with $MgCl_2$).

   1 μl 2 mM dATP.

   0.25 μl TAQ polymerase (5U).

   (b) Incubate the reaction at 72 °C for 30 min.

3. Digest the respective entry vector with XcmI for 3 h at 37 °C. Purify the vector as described above.

4. Set up a ligation using 20 ng of the digested vector and the threefold molar amount of the A-tailed insert. The standard approach discussed above has also been successfully applied.

5. Incubate the ligation overnight at 16 °C and continue as described above.

3.1.3 Cloning Oligonucleotides into Entry Vectors

The protocol for single-oligo duplex cloning is derived from the Life Technologies website. It is a part of the shRNA cloning procedure of the BLOCK-it shRNA expression vectors (*see* **Note 6**). Oligos have to be double stranded for cloning; thus two oligos have to be ordered for each fragment (Fig. 3b). One contains the forward 5′–3′ sequence and the other one has to be the reverse complement. Furthermore, in order to facilitate subcloning, the BamHI and KpnI overhangs have to be included. Based on the orientation of the cuts from the enzymes, both overhangs must be included in the forward oligo. The reverse oligo contains only the reverse complement of the proper DNA fragment.

**Cloning
of a Single-Oligo Duplex**

1. Dilute the ordered oligos to 200 μM with H_2O (*see* **Note 6**).
2. Mix the following reaction:

    5 μl Oligo forward.

    5 μl Oligo reverse.

    2 μl 10× Oligo annealing buffer (OAB).

    8 μl H2O.
3. Heat to 95 °C in a heating block for 4 min.
4. Let the reaction cool down on the bench for at least 30 min.
5. Dilute the annealed oligos 1:100 in H_2O to obtain dilution A (*see* **Note 8**).
6. Dilute dilution A 1:50 in 1× OAB (1 μl dilution A + 44 μl H_2O + 5 μl 10× OAB) to obtain dilution B.
7. Dilution B is the final dilution for the ligation reaction:

    1 μl vector (digested with BamHI/KpnI, 20 ng/μl, DO NOT dephosphorylate!).

    7 μl Dilution B.

    1 μl T4 ligase (5U).

    1 μl T4 ligase buffer.
8. Continue with ligation and transformation as described above.

**Cloning
of Multiple-Oligo Sets**

1. Dissolve oligos to get 200 pmol/μl.
2. Mix this reaction with each oligo separately to phosphorylate the oligos:

    8 μl Oligo stock.

    1 μl T4 ligase buffer.

    1 μl T4 polynucleotide kinase.
3. Incubate for 1 h at 37 °C, and then heat inactivate for 15 min at 75 °C.
4. Set up the following reaction:

    5 μl Oligo 1.

    5 μl Oligo 2.

    2 μl 10× OAB.

    8 μl H2O.
5. Continue with standard oligo annealing procedure for all fragments to obtain OA1 and OA2.
6. Cut 2 μg of the vector backbone with BamHI and KpnI as described above.
7. Purify the cut vector from the agarose gel and elute in 30 μl H_2O.
8. Dephosphorylate the vector backbone:

    30 μl Vector.

3.5 µl 10× FastDigest buffer.

1 µl FastAP alkaline phosphatase.

7. Incubate for 25 min at 37 °C, and then heat inactivate for 15 min at 75 °C.

8. Ligate the following reaction:

1 µl Vector.

5 µl OA1.

5 µl OA2.

1.3 µl 10× T4 ligase buffer.

1 µl T4 ligase (5U).

9. Incubate for 2 h at RT.

10. Continue with the standard transformation and colony identification described above.

3.1.4 Site-Directed Mutagenesis Using Golden Gate Cloning

We established vectors to assemble PCR products via Golden Gate cloning that contain flanking BamHI and KpnI sites for cloning of the assembled DNA fragment to the entry vectors (Fig. 3c). The primers for the PCR reaction need to contain flanking BsaI sites with matching overhangs. This means that four consecutive bases can be simultaneously changed between two PCR products. The flanking PCR products need to contain BsaI sites that allow ligation to the pSdM vectors: Append to forward primer: NNNN-GGTCTC-A-CGTG; append to reverse primer: NNNN-GGTCTC-G-CGAC. We routinely use the proofreading Q5 polymerase with a standard PCR reaction to amplify the fragments.

1. Design and order the primers according to the primer design guidelines (Fig. 3c).

2. Prepare a standard PCR reaction to amplify the fragments.

3. Purify the PCR reactions from an agarose gel.

4. Use 20 fm of each PCR product and the pSdM vector for a Golden Gate assembly:

1 µl of each PCR product (diluted to 20 fm/µl).

1 µl 10× Fast Digest buffer.

1 µl 10× T4 ligase buffer.

1 µl 10 mM ATP.

0.5 µl BsaI.

0.5 µl T4 ligase HC (30U).

Adjust to 20 µl with H2O.

5. Transform 3–10 µl of the assembly as described above. Plate on kanamycin plates supplemented with IPTG and X-Gal.

3.2 Golden Gate Reaction

1. Prepare a 20 fm/μl dilution for each vector (entry vectors and the destination vector). Take care to vortex it well and re-measure the dilution with the Nanodrop (*see* **Note 9**).

2. Assemble the following reaction:

   1 μl of each vector (max. 9 μl).

   1 μl Fast Digest buffer.

   1 μl T4 ligase buffer.

   1 μl ATP (*see* **Note 10**).

   0.5 μl BsaI (*see* **Note 11**).

   0.5 μl T4 ligase HC (30U).

   Add 20 μl with H2O.

   (*see* **Note 12**.)

3. Incubate the reaction using the following cycling conditions:

   37 °C for 30 min (BsaI can cut the DNA efficiently).

   15 °C for 20 min (T4 ligase can ligate the 4 bp overhangs more efficiently because of higher annealing efficiency).

   Repeat 5–10×.

   (*see* **Note 13**.)

4. Continue with the standard transformation and colony identification described above (*see* **Note 14**).

3.3 Further Use of the Assembled Construct

3.3.1 Multisite Gateway Cloning

1. Use 0.5 μl of each vector (20 fmol) with 0.5 μl of the LR Clonase II Plus (*see* **Note 15**).

2. Incubate the reactions at 25 °C for 16 h in a PCR machine without lid heating.

3. Add 2 μl H$_2$O, mix the entire reaction with 25 μl competent cells, and proceed with the transformation as described above.

3.3.2 Golden Gate Cloning Assembly via XcmI Back to pEVs

If the pShuffle vector was used as the destination vector for the Golden Gate assembly, then the assembled DNA fragment can be released from the vector backbone with XcmI and ligated back into an entry vector to assemble it with additional fragments.

4 Notes

1. It is possible to skip the generation of entry vectors completely with a PCR- or oligo-cloning-based approach. For that, the flanking BsaI sites from the corresponding entry vector have to be attached at the 5′ and 3′ end. In some cases, this can save time. However, it also comes with multiple disadvantages. First, the DNA fragment in an entry vector is defined and should be sequenced. The exact sequence of the PCR reaction

or annealed oligos do not necessarily fit the expected sequence based on mutations introduced during the manufacturing process. Additionally, purified PCR products as well as annealed oligos are not as stable as proper entry vectors. Finally, the recurring multiple cloning site in the entry vectors allows shuffling of the DNA fragment between entry vectors. By circumventing the entry vectors, one has to order new oligos and prepare the oligo annealing or the PCR reaction again.

2. After the entry vector digestion a single band must be cut out; multiple bands indicate improper digestion.

3. For most applications, we use a standard amount of purified insert. We routinely use the 5U T4 ligase from NEB with the supplemented buffer. Thus, a standard reaction is 1 μl of the vector (20 ng) and 7 μl of the purified insert (standardized amount), together with 1 μl of the 10× T4 ligation buffer and 1 μl of the T4 ligase (5U).

4. The ligations and all subsequent reactions can be transformed into standard *E. coli* lab strains following standard protocols. We routinely use chemical competent cells from the MachT1 strain (Thermo Scientific/Life technologies).

5. For the competent cells we use, IPTG induction is not necessary. If lacI+ *E. coli* are used, supplement the plates with 40 μl X-Gal and 40 μl IPTG.

6. Cloning of longer DNA fragments with multiple-oligo pairs is especially useful to clone fragments with a length of 120–300 bp since such long oligos cannot be synthesized and the PCR reaction of such small fragments is in our experience often difficult to purify and to use for further cloning. Design the oligos to obtain matching overhangs after proper fusion of the annealed DNA fragments. We routinely order desalted oligos without further purification. We observe only very limited numbers of mutations in these primers. We have successfully cloned a single-oligo duplex with a length of 100 bp using this method.

7. The high oligo concentration of 200 μM is necessary for the annealing.

8. Optionally the annealing can be checked on a 4% agarose gel. Load 3 μl of dilution A on the gel. For a negative control, mix 0.5 μl of the oligos with 199 μl H_2O. However, this protocol is very robust so that we usually skip this step.

9. It is crucial that the entry vectors are purified as well as stored and diluted in pure H_2O since any buffer components might inhibit the Golden Gate assembly.

10. The ligation buffer is supplemented with ATP, which is degraded by freeze-thaw cycles. Thus, we prepare small aliquots of the buffer.

11. The quality of the BsaI (Eco31I) enzyme is crucial for the efficiency of the assembly. In our experience, the FastDigest version of Eco31I (Thermo Scientific/Life Technologies) shows maximum efficiency. Store the enzyme at –20 °C, prepare aliquots, and only use it for maximum 6 months.

12. Extra ATP is added although the 10× T4 ligation buffer also contains ATP. Having two sources of ATP increases the likelihood that enough ATP is present even if some degradation might have occurred in the buffer or the ATP stock solution. Beware not to add more ATP since too much ATP inhibits the ligation reaction. Additionally, the T4 ligase buffer includes DTT, which helps to maintain protein activity.

13. Internal BsaI sites in the inserts can be problematic for the assembly, since these parts will be cut as well. However, if the generated overhang is not compatible with overhangs of any entry vector or destination vector used in the assembly the reaction can still work. These parts will be ligated again in another re-ligation step by adding 1 μl of T4 DNA ligase (5 U) after the cycling incubation of the Golden Gate reaction. Incubating the reaction at RT for 20 min should ligate all potentially cut BsaI sites in the assembly.

14. In rare cases, a complete backbone from an entry vector can be ligated into the final assembly; hence the colonies would appear white but are false positives. To discard false-positive colonies the same colony can be picked in both LB-kanamycin and LB-ampicillin. The LB-kanamycin cultures can be trashed if the corresponding Amp culture grows as well.

15. We usually successfully use only ¼ of the suggested amount of vector and LR clonase for the Multisite Gateway reaction.

References

1. Kirchmaier S, Lust K, Wittbrodt J (2013) Golden GATEway cloning—a combinatorial approach to generate fusion and recombination constructs. PLoS One 8:e76117. doi:10.1371/journal.pone.0076117

2. Engler C, Gruetzner R, Kandzia R, Marillonnet S (2009) Golden gate shuffling: a one-pot DNA shuffling method based on type IIs restriction enzymes. PLoS One 4:e5553. doi:10.1371/journal.pone.0005553

3. Curtis MD, Curtis MD, Grossniklaus U (2015) A gateway cloning vector set for high-throughput functional analysis of genes in planta. Plant Physiol 133:462–469. doi:10.1104/pp.103.027979.specific

4. Kwan KM, Fujimoto E, Grabher C et al (2007) The Tol2kit: a multisite gateway-based construction kit for Tol2 transposon transgenesis constructs. Dev Dyn 236:3088–3099. doi:10.1002/dvdy.21343

5. Zeiser E, Frøkjær-Jensen C, Jorgensen E, Ahringer J (2011) MosSCI and gateway compatible plasmid toolkit for constitutive and inducible expression of transgenes in the C. elegans germline. PLoS One 6:e20082. doi:10.1371/journal.pone.0020082

6. Distel M, Wullimann MF, Ko RW (2009) Optimized Gal4 genetics for permanent gene expression mapping in zebrafish. Proc Natl Acad Sci U S A 106:13365–13370

Chapter 13

Gene Deletion by Synthesis in Yeast

Jinsil Kim, Dong-Uk Kim, and Kwang-Lae Hoe

Abstract

Targeted gene deletion is a useful tool for understanding the function of a gene and its protein product. We have developed an efficient and robust gene deletion approach in yeast that employs oligonucleotide-based gene synthesis. This approach requires a deletion cassette composed of three modules: a central 1397-bp KanMX4 selection marker module and two 366-bp gene-specific flanking modules. The invariable KanMX4 module can be used in combination with different pairs of flanking modules targeting different genes. The two flanking modules consist of both sequences unique to each cassette (chromosomal homologous regions and barcodes) and those common to all deletion constructs (artificial linkers and restriction enzyme sites). Oligonucleotides for each module and junction regions are designed using the BatchBlock2Oligo program and are synthesized on a 96-well basis. The oligonucleotides are ligated into a single deletion cassette by ligase chain reaction, which is then amplified through two rounds of nested PCR to obtain sufficient quantities for yeast transformation. After removal of the artificial linkers, the deletion cassettes are transformed into wild-type diploid fission yeast SP286 cells. Verification of correct clone and gene deletion is achieved by performing check PCR and tetrad analysis. This method with proven effectiveness, as evidenced by a high success rate of gene deletion, can be potentially applicable to create systematic gene deletion libraries in a variety of yeast species.

Key words Yeast, Targeted gene deletion, Deletion cassette, Artificial sequence linker, Gene synthesis, Ligase chain reaction

1 Introduction

Gene deletion is a useful approach to study the function of a particular gene and its protein product(s). One of the successfully used methods for gene deletion involves the insertion of an extraneous DNA fragment into the coding region of a target gene, which, in most cases, results in disruption of its reading frame, causing the production of a non-functional protein. Alternatively, the insertion may lead to replacement of the entire endogenous coding region with a selectable marker, thereby generating a null allele. In yeast, which has a highly efficient homologous recombination system, gene deletion can be achieved in a targeted manner through a one-step approach. In this approach, a linear DNA fragment (a deletion cassette)

Randall A. Hughes (ed.), *Synthetic DNA: Methods and Protocols*, Methods in Molecular Biology, vol. 1472,
DOI 10.1007/978-1-4939-6343-0_13, © Springer Science+Business Media New York 2017

containing a selectable marker gene with regions homologous to the sequence flanking the gene to be deleted (hereinafter referred to as chromosomal homologous regions, CHRs) integrates into the corresponding genomic locus, replacing the target gene [1–3]. The deletion cassette also has a pair of molecular barcodes (unique nucleotide sequences specific to each cassette) located upstream and downstream of the selectable marker, allowing later identification of each resulting deletion mutant strain [3–6]. The CHRs can be as short as 30–50 bp for *Saccharomyces cerevisiae* (*S. cerevisiae*) and 80–100 bp for *Schizosaccharomyces pombe* (*S. pombe*), making it possible to generate deletion cassettes by polymerase chain reaction (PCR) without the need for cloning steps [7]. The selectable marker gene consists of completely heterologous DNA to limit homologous recombination to the CHRs [8]. The *kan*[r] gene, which confers resistance to the antibiotic geneticin (G418), is the first heterologous dominant selectable marker used for gene disruption [8]. This marker gene has been a useful tool in the construction of a collection of over 6,000 *S. cerevisiae* deletion strains that can serve as a valuable resource of single-gene-loss-of-function mutants [6–9]. Similarly, a genome-wide single-gene deletion mutant library has been generated for the fission yeast *S. pombe* [5, 7], expanding the scope of genetic functional analysis of eukaryotic genes (*see* **Note 1**).

The efficiency of gene deletion is known to increase with the length of the CHRs, but lengthening the CHRs can concomitantly cause an increase in the difficulty of cassette preparation [3, 10, 11]. In *S. cerevisiae*, deletion cassettes with ~50 bp CHRs were generated by sequential PCR reactions and successfully used for the deletion of the majority of target genes [3, 6, 9]. However, in *S. pombe*, the same strategy was applicable to 31 % (1,515/4,836) of the deletion mutant library with the remaining two thirds (3,321/4,836) constructed using deletion cassettes with longer (~250 bp) CHRs [3, 5] prepared by block PCR [10, 12–14]. One disadvantage of block PCR is that it requires purification of PCR products by gel elution, which is an elaborate and technically challenging procedure. In order to alleviate this technical difficulty, a novel gene synthesis method was developed and used to generate systematic gene deletions in *S. pombe* [5]. Although this method provided increased convenience in the preparation of deletion cassettes, it still needs to be refined in several aspects to achieve maximum efficiency and accuracy in targeted deletion.

Here, we provide an optimized protocol for the gene synthesis method used to construct gene deletion libraries in *S. pombe* [3, 5], which involves design and synthesis of oligonucleotides for a deletion cassette, ligation of synthetic oligonucleotides through ligase chain reaction (LCR), amplification of the LCR product using artificial sequence linker-specific primers, yeast transformation with the deletion cassette, verification of correct clone and gene deletion by PCR, and tetrad analysis. The protocol provided here is potentially applicable to other yeast species.

2 Materials

2.1 Deletion Cassette and Oligonucleotide Design

The deletion cassette, which is 2,129 bp long, is divided into three modules: a 1,397-bp invariable kanamycin resistance (KanMX4) module and a pair of 366-bp variable gene-specific flanking modules (Fig. 1a). The KanMX4 module contains the *kanr* open reading frame (ORF) of the *Escherichia coli* (*E. coli*) Tn903 transposon fused to promoter and terminator sequences from the TEF gene of the yeast *Ashbya gossypii* (*see* **Note 2**). The gene-specific 5′ and 3′ CHRs (each with a length of 250 bp) consist of sequences from the promoter region upstream of the ATG start codon and the terminator region downstream of the stop codon(s), respectively, of the gene to be deleted. In the 46-bp 5′ and 3′ artificial linker regions, there are binding sites for two pairs of primer for two rounds of nested PCR (L1-F/L1-R and L2-F/L2-R) and Eco31I restriction enzyme sites (5′-GGTCTCN-3′) for removal of the artificial linkers before yeast transformation (Fig. 1b). The 70-bp barcode region contains a central 20-mer up-tag or down-tag with flanking gaps and universal primer-binding sites (U1-F/U2-R or D1-F/D2-R) for PCR amplification of the barcode (Fig. 1c).

For oligonucleotide design, Internet connection, web browser software, and Microsoft Excel or other spreadsheet software are needed. The entire set of oligonucleotides for gene synthesis is designed using the BatchBlock2Oligo program, which incorporates two previously used algorithms named Block2Oligo and iBlocks2Assembly [5]. The BatchBlock2Oligo program can be accessed at http://pombe.kaist.ac.kr/block2oligo/batch_block2oligo.pl. Oligonucleotides can be synthesized on a 96-well basis.

2.2 Ligase Chain Reaction

1. Oligonucleotides.
2. 10 mM Adenosine-5′-triphosphate (ATP).
3. 10 U/μl T4 polynucleotide kinase.
4. 10× T4 polynucleotide kinase buffer: 700 mM Tris–HCl, 100 mM MgCl$_2$, 50 mM dithiothreitol (DTT), pH 7.6 at 25 °C.
5. 20 U/μl *Thermus filiformis* (*Tfi*) DNA ligase (Bioneer, Alameda, CA, USA) (*see* **Note 3**).
6. 10× *Tfi* DNA ligase reaction buffer: 300 mM Tris–HCl, pH 8.3, 250 mM KCl, 50 mM MgCl$_2$, 5 mM β-Nicotinamide adenine dinucleotide (NAD).
7. Sterile ddH$_2$O.
8. 96-Well microplate.
9. Thermocycler.

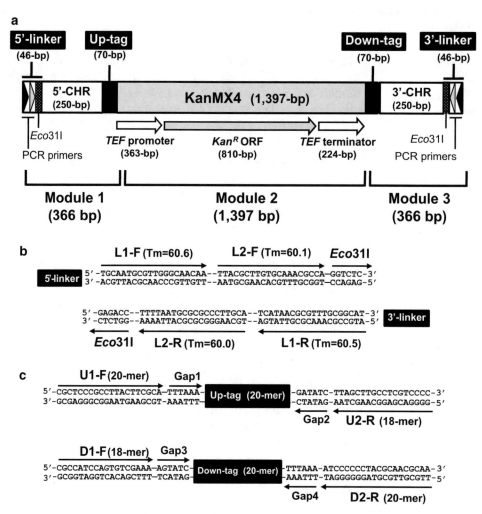

Fig. 1 Schematic diagram of a deletion cassette. (**a**) A deletion cassette with a length of 2129 bp is composed of three modules: modules 1 and 3 containing an artificial linker, a CHR, and an up-tag or down-tag and module 2 consisting of the *kan*^D1-F/D-R ORF flanked by the TEF promoter and terminator. (**b**) Structure and sequence of artificial linkers. The 5′ and 3′ linker regions harbor two sets of primer-binding sites (L1-F/L1-R and L2-F/L2-R) for nested PCR and Eco31I restriction enzyme sites. (**c**) Structure and sequence of molecular barcodes. The barcode region comprises a 20-mer up-tag or down-tag flanked by universal primer-binding sites (U1-F/U2-R for the up-tag or D1-F/D2-R for the down-tag) with in-between gap sequences, which are inserted for efficient PCR amplification of the barcodes (reproduced from [3] with permission from Elsevier)

2.3   Nested PCR

1. 2.5 U/μl *Pfu* DNA polymerase (Bioneer, Alameda, CA, USA).

2. 10× *Pfu* polymerase buffer: 200 mM Tris–HCl, 100 mM KCl, 100 mM $(NH_4)_2SO_4$, 20 mM $MgSO_4$, 1% Triton X-100, 1 mg/ml acetylated BSA, pH 8.8.

3. Artificial linker primer pairs: L1-F/ L1-R for the first round nested PCR, L2-F/L2-R for the second round nested PCR (Fig. 1b), 100 pmol/μl each.

4. Sequencing primers that bind to the artificial linker regions.

5. 10 mM each dNTP.

6. Sterile ddH$_2$O.

7. 96-Well microplate.

8. Thermocycler.

2.4 Yeast Transformation

Yeast transformation is carried out using the lithium acetate method described in [15].

1. Eco31I: 10 U/µl.

2. 10× Eco31I reaction buffer: 100 mM Tris–HCl (pH 7.5), 100 mM MgCl$_2$, 500 mM NaCl, 1 mg/ml BSA.

3. Sterile ddH$_2$O.

4. YE medium (1 l): 5 g Yeast extract and 30 g glucose in ddH$_2$O. Autoclave.

5. 1/2 YE medium (1 l): 2.5 g Yeast extract and 15 g glucose in ddH$_2$O. Autoclave. Or dilute 500 ml YE medium to 1 l with ddH$_2$O.

6. Minimal (+ uracil and leucine) (1 l): 3 g Potassium hydrogen phthalate, 2.2 g Na$_2$HPO$_4$, 5 g NH$_4$Cl, 20 g D-glucose, 20 ml 50× salt stock, 1 ml 1000× vitamin stock, 0.1 ml 10,000× mineral stock, 300 mg/l each of uracil and leucine. Autoclave. For the compositions of salt, vitamin, and mineral stocks, see below or [15].
   50× salt stock: 52.5 g/l MgCl$_2$·6H$_2$O, 0.735 mg/l CaCl$_2$·2H$_2$O, 50 g/l KCl, 2 g/l Na$_2$SO$_4$.
   1000× vitamin stock: 1 g/l pantothenic acid, 10 g/l nicotinic acid, 10 g/l inositol, 10 mg/l biotin.
   10,000× mineral stock: 5 g/l H$_3$BO$_3$, 4 g/l MnSO$_4$, 4 g/l ZnSO$_4$ 7H$_2$O, 2 g/l FeCl$_3$·6H$_2$O, 0.4 g/l molybdic acid, 1 g/l KI, 0.4 g/l CuSO$_4$·5H$_2$O, 10 g/l citric acid.

7. YEUL medium (1 l): 5 g Yeast extract, 30 g glucose, 250 mg/l each of uracil and leucine in ddH$_2$O. Autoclave.

8. 0.1 M Lithium acetate solution, pH 4.9 (1 l): Dissolve 51 g of lithium acetate dihydrate in 1 l of ddH$_2$O, sterilize by autoclaving for 15 min, and store at room temperature.

9. 50% (w/v) PEG 4000: Dissolve 100 g of polyethylene glycol (PEG) 4000 in a final volume of 200 ml ddH$_2$O. Autoclave to sterilize.

10. YEUL + G418: Dissolve 40 mg geneticin/G418 in 2 ml sterile ddH$_2$O and add to 400 ml warm (<60 °C) YEUL medium + 20 g/l agar to obtain a final concentration of 100 µg/ml G418. Use freshly prepared plates.

11. Geneticin (G418).

12. SP286 (*h+/h + ade6-M210/ade6-M216, ura4-D18/ura4-D18, leu1-32/leu1-32*) cells.

13. Sterile microcentrifuge tubes.

14. Sterile 50 and 250 ml Erlenmeyer flasks.

15. Water bath.

16. Microcentrifuge.

17. Shaking incubator.

2.5 Check PCR

1. *Taq* DNA polymerase: 5 U/μl.

2. 10× PCR reaction buffer without MgCl$_2$: 100 mM Tris–HCl, 400 mM KCl, pH 9.0.

3. 20 mM MgCl$_2$.

4. 2.5 mM each dNTP.

5. PCR primers: Four gene-specific primers (cp5 and cp3, cp5i and cp3i) and four KanMX module-binding primers (Fig. 2). The sequence of the KanMX module-binding primers are shown below:

Name	Sequence
cp-N1	5′-CGTCTGTGAGGGGAGCGTTT-3′
cp-N10	5′-GATGTGAGAACTGTATCCTAGCAAG-3′
cp-C1	5′-TGATTTTGATGACGAGCGTAAT-3′
cp-C3	5′-GGCTGGCCTGTTGAACAAGTCTGGA-3′

To find the sequence of the cp5 and cp3 primers for a deletion mutant from the *S. pombe* genome-wide deletion mutant library [5], go to http://pombe.kaist.ac.kr/nbtsupp, enter a gene or systematic name in the "Interactive queries" search box and click

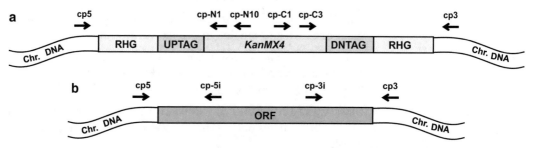

Fig. 2 Verification of deletion mutants by check PCR. (**a**) Check that PCR is performed using two gene-specific primers (cp5 and cp3) and four KanMX module-binding primers (cp-N1, cp-N10, cp-C1, and cp-C3). The cp5 and cp3 primers are located from 400 to 600 bp upstream of the start codon and 400 to 600 bp downstream of the stop codon, respectively, of a target gene. Correctly sized products are produced only for successful deletion mutants when PCR is performed using different combinations of these primers, cp5/cp-N1 (or cp-N10) and the cp3/cp-C1 (or cp-C3). (**b**) For unsuccessful deletion mutants, another round of PCR is performed using cp5i and cp3i primers binding within the CDS region to check if the coding sequence of a target gene is still present (reproduced from [5] with permission from Nature Publishing Group)

the "GO" button. On the next page, click "View Mapping," and it will lead you to the page containing the sequence and position of cp5 and cp3 primers and expected check PCR product sizes.

6. Sterile ddH$_2$O.

7. 10× TAE buffer (Sigma, T8280): Bring to 1× by adding 100–900 ml ddH$_2$O.

8. Agarose, loading dye, and nucleic acid stain suitable for gel electrophoresis.

9. 1 kb DNA ladder.

2.6 Tetrad Analysis

Tetrad analysis is carried out using the method described in [15].

1. pON177 plasmid [16].

2. Minimal (+ adenine and leucine) plates (1 l): 3 g Potassium hydrogen phthalate, 2.2 g Na$_2$HPO$_4$, 5 g NH$_4$Cl, 20 g D-glucose, 20 ml 50× salt stock, 1 ml 1,000× vitamin stock, 0.1 ml 10,000× mineral stock, 300 mg/l each of adenine and leucine. Add 20 g/l agar and autoclave. For the compositions of salt, vitamin, and mineral stocks, *see* Subheading 2.4 or [15].

3. YES plates: 5 g/l Yeast extract, 30 g/l glucose, 250 mg/l each of adenine, uracil, and leucine, and 20 g/l agar in ddH$_2$O. Autoclave.

4. YES + G418 plates: Dissolve 40 mg geneticin/G418 in 2 ml sterile ddH$_2$O and add to 400 ml warm (<60 °C) YES medium + 20 g/l agar to obtain a final concentration of 100 μg/ml G418. Use freshly prepared plates.

5. Microscopic manipulator (Singer MSM, Somerset, England).

3 Methods

3.1 Deletion Cassette and Oligonucleotide Design

A deletion cassette is composed of sequences that are unique to each cassette (CHR and barcode sequences) as well as those that are common to all deletion constructs (linker, restriction enzyme site, and KanMX4 sequences). The unique 20-mer barcode (up-tag and down-tag) sequences are generated using a BioPerl-based program on the basis of the following criteria: melting temperature (Tm) = 60 °C, no cross-hybridization, no secondary structures, and no homology to genomic sequences (*see* **Note 4**) [5].

To design oligonucleotides for deletion cassette construction, the nucleotide sequences of the cassette components are merged in three sets—BLOCK 1 (5′-linker, Eco31I, 5′-CHR, up-tag), BLOCK 2 (KanMX4), and BLOCK 3 (down-tag, 3′-CHR, Eco31I, 3′-linker). The sequences in these BLOCKs are used as query sequences for the BatchBlock2Oligo program (http://pombe.kaist.ac.kr/block2oligo/batch_block2oligo.pl), which outputs a list of oligonucleotides covering the three BLOCKS as well as those bridging the BLOCKS. A major basic principle for oligonucleotide design is to minimize Tm differences. A Tm of 60 ± 3 °C is considered as a first parameter, with the Tm calculated using the nearest-neighbor thermodynamics [17]. In addition, an oligonucleotide length of 25–35 mers is regarded as an important factor to minimize errors in chemical synthesis [3]. The process of designing oligonucleotides using the BatchBlock2Oligo program is described in detail in the program website under "Batch block2oligo Tutorial."

As an illustrative example, the oligonucleotide set used for deletion of the dynein light chain Dlc1 gene (*dlc1*, SPAC1805.08) is shown in Fig. 3 [3]. The total number of oligonucleotides generated to construct the *dlc1*deletion cassette was 147 (25 each for modules 1 and 3 + 93 for module 2 + 4 for junction regions between the modules, Fig. 3a) [3]. The oligonucleotide set for modules 1 and 3 includes terminal oligonucleotides for making the ends of the deletion cassette blunt (Fig. 3b). The majority of oligonucleotides were ~29 mer long with the terminal and junction oligonucleotides being 12–16 and 20–30 mer long, respectively (Fig. 3b) [3].

3.2 Ligase Chain Reaction

The oligonucleotides synthesized are assembled into a single deletion cassette through LCR after their 5′ ends are phosphorylated. Provided below is a 96-well format protocol.

1. To phosphorylate the 5′ ends of oligonucleotides using T4 polynucleotide kinase, prepare the following reaction mixture:

Reagent	Final concentration	Volume (μl)
Oligonucleotides (20 pmol each/reaction)	0.4 pmol/μl each	29
10× T4 polynucleotide kinase reaction buffer	1×	5
T4 polynucleotide kinase (10 U/μl)	1 U/μl	5
10 mM ATP	1.6 mM	8
Total volume		47

2. Incubate the phosphorylation reaction at 37 °C for 5 h in a thermocycler.

3. Add additional 3 μl T4 polynucleotide kinase to the reaction from the previous step and incubate at 37 °C for another 5 h.

4. After the second 5-h incubation, set up the following LCR reaction mixture:

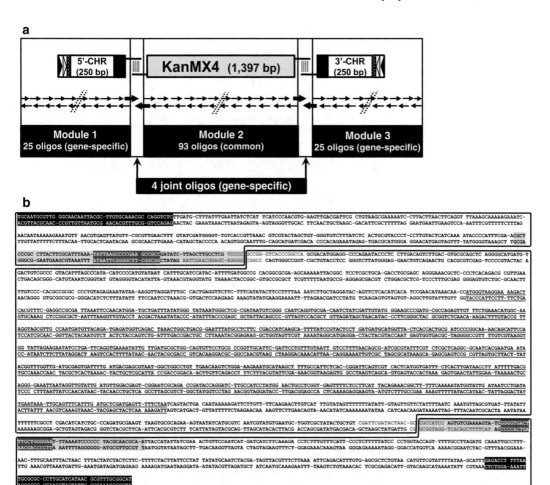

Fig. 3 Oligonucleotides used for *dlc1* (SPAC1805.08) deletion cassette construction. (**a**) Schematic diagram of the *dlc1* deletion cassette showing the number of oligonucleotides used for construction of each module and the junction regions. (**b**) Sequences of 147 *dlc1* deletion cassette oligonucleotides. Each module is marked with a *box* and different oligonucleotides are separated by *spaces*. *Dashes* represent gaps inserted to obtain optimal alignment. The artificial linkers and the barcode regions are highlighted in *black* and *gray*, respectively, with the sequences highlighted in *blue* within the barcode regions in modules 1 and 3 representing the up-tag and the down-tag, respectively. The terminal oligonucleotide sequences at both ends of the deletion cassette are shown in *yellow*. The oligonucleotides underlined in module 2 correspond to the KanMX4 ORF, which is flanked by the non-underlined TEF promoter (5′) and terminator (3′) sequences. Represented in red are the junction oligonucleotides between modules 1 and 2 and modules 2 and 3 (reproduced from [3] with permission from Elsevier)

Reagent	Final concentration	Volume (μl)
Phosphorylated oligonucleotides (8.7 pmol each/reaction)	0.29 pmol/μl each	24
10× *Tfi* DNA ligase reaction buffer	1×	3
Tfi DNA ligase (20 U/μl)	2 U/μl	3
Total volume		30

5. Incubate the LCR reaction mixture in a thermocycler using the conditions shown below:

Denaturation	95 °C	5 min
Ligation	50–60 °C	5 min
Cycles	40	

It is critical to find an optimal ligation temperature for LCR in order to obtain maximum yield of ligated products. As shown in Fig. 4a, b, the yields of the deletion cassettes after two rounds of nested PCR greatly differ depending on the ligation temperature used (*see* **Note 5**) [3].

3.3 Nested PCR

The yield of the resulting LCR products (deletion cassettes without nicks) is extremely low and therefore the cassettes should be amplified through two consecutive rounds of nested PCR to obtain sufficient amount of DNA for yeast transformation.

1. Prepare the first-round nested PCR reaction mixture as follows:

Reagent	Final concentration	Volume (µl)
Template DNA: LCR products		1
10× *Pfu* polymerase buffer	1×	2
Pfu polymerase (2.5 U/µl)	0.125 U/µl	1
Artificial linker primer pair (L1-F and L1-R, 100 pmol/µl each)	2.5 pmol/µl each	1
dNTPs (each at 10 mM)	0.25 mM each	0.5
ddH₂O		14.5
Total volume		20

2. Perform the PCR reaction using the following conditions:

Initial incubation	94 °C	2 min
Denaturation	94 °C	30 s
Annealing	60 °C	30 s
Polymerization	72 °C	2 min
Final incubation	72 °C	5 min
Cycles	35	

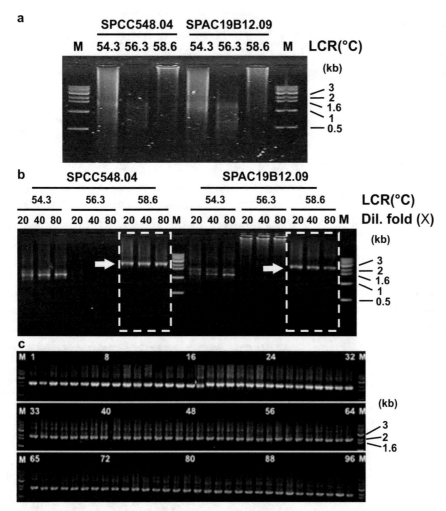

Fig. 4 Ligase chain reaction (LCR) and nested PCR for assembly and amplification of deletion cassettes targeting *urm1* (SPCC548.04) and *srp14* (SPAC19B12.09). (**a**) The LCR products ligated at 54.3, 56.3, and 58.6 °C were amplified by the first-round nested PCR, which yielded no discrete bands on an agarose gel. *Lanes* named *M* represent a 1 kb DNA ladder. (**b**) Diluted first-round nested PCR products (20-, 40-, and 80-fold) were amplified by the second-round nested PCR. Amplification of the LCR products ligated at 58.6 °C only produced correctly sized bands (*dotted boxes, white arrows*). (**c**) Gel electrophoresis of the second-round nested PCR products of a batch of 96 deletion cassettes. The two rounds of nested PCR resulted in sufficient quantities (>1 μg) of deletion cassettes for transformation. *Lanes* named *M* represent a 1 kb DNA ladder (reproduced from [3] with permission from Elsevier)

3. Prepare the following second-round nested PCR reaction mixture:

Reagent	Final concentration	Volume (μl)
Template DNA: first-round nested PCR products		1
10× *Pfu* polymerase buffer	1×	2

Reagent	Final concentration	Volume (µl)
Pfu polymerase (2.5 U/µl)	0.125 U/µl	1
Artificial linker primer pair (L2-F and L2-R, 100 pmol/µl each)	2.5 pmol/µl each	1
dNTPs (each at 10 mM)	0.25 mM each	0.5
ddH$_2$O		14.5
Total volume		20

4. Carry out the second-round nested PCR reaction using the identical cycling conditions described above (**step 2**).

5. Verify the sequence of the amplified PCR products (deletion cassettes) by dideoxy sequencing using primers annealing to the linker regions.

3.4 Yeast Transformation (According to [15])

1. Before transformation, set up the following Eco31I digestion reaction to remove the artificial linkers from the nested PCR products and incubate at 37 °C for 3–6 h (*see* **Note 6**):

Reagent	Final concentration	Volume (µl)
Second-round nested PCR products		20
10× Eco31I reaction buffer	1×	5
Eco31I restriction enzyme (10 U/µl)	0.6 U/µl	3
ddH$_2$O		22
Total volume		50

2. After 3–6 h, incubate the above reaction mixture at 65 °C for 20 min to heat inactivate Eco31I (*see* **Note 7**).

3. Start a pre-culture from a single colony in 3 ml minimal (YE + ura, leu) medium at 30 °C for 12 h on a shaker (*see* **Note 8**).

4. After 12 h, inoculate a 10 ml culture in YES medium from the pre-culture at a cell density of OD$_{600}$ = 0.2 in 250 ml Erlenmeyer flask and grow to OD$_{600}$ = 0.5 at 30 °C with continuous shaking (*see* **Note 9**).

5. Harvest cells by centrifugation at 735 × *g* for 3 min at room temperature.

6. Add 40 ml sterile distilled water to the cell pellet, resuspend by repeated inversions, and harvest the cells as above.

7. Repeat the cell wash with 40 ml 0.1 M lithium acetate solution as above, spin, and resuspend the cells in 0.5–1.0 ml lithium acetate solution at a density of about 1 × 10^9 cells/ml. Make

100 μl aliquots in sterile microcentrifuge tubes and incubate for 40 min at 30 °C. Cells sediment at this stage.

8. Add 20–30 μl Eco31l-digested deletion cassette DNA and mix by gently vortexing. And then, add 290 μl of 50% (w/v) PEG4000 solution pre-warmed to 30 °C and vortex. Incubate for 40 min at 30 °C.

9. Heat shock at 42 °C for 15 min. Cool the tubes to room temperature for 10 min.

10. Harvest the cells by centrifugation (microcentrifuge at $1300 \times g$ for 2 min). Remove the supernatant by aspiration. Resuspend the cells in 1 ml of 1/2 YE medium by pipetting up and down.

11. Transfer the suspension to a 50 ml flask and dilute with 9 ml of 1/2 YE medium. Incubate at 30 °C overnight.

12. Centrifuge the cells and resuspend in 3 ml of 1/2 YE medium.

13. Plate aliquots (50 μl) onto YEUL agar plates with 100 μg/ml G418 and incubate at 30 °C until appearance of colonies (about 3–4 days).

3.5 Check PCR

Check PCR must be performed to confirm that the disruption cassette has integrated correctly and replaced the intended target gene. The primer combinations cp5/cp-N1 (or cp-N10) and the cp3/cp-C1 (or cp-C3) will generate a specific PCR product only if the deletion cassette has integrated at the correct location (Fig. 2a).

1. Colony-purify the yeast transformants on YES + G418 agar plates. For PCR, always use freshly grown cells (no more than 2 days old).

2. To obtain cells for check PCR, lightly touch the surface of a yeast colony with a yellow pipette tip, resuspend in 200 μl sterile ddH₂O, and centrifuge cells down at $8200 \times g$ for 30 s.

3. Repeat the above step, aspirate the suspension, and resuspend cells in 50 μl sterile ddH₂O.

4. Set up the following check PCR reaction mixture:

Reagent	Final concentration	Volume (μl)
Template DNA: suspension from **step 3**		1
10× PCR reaction buffer	1×	2
Primer pairs: cp5/cp-N1 (or cp-N10) and cp3/cp-C1 (or cp-C3), 100 pmol/μl each	5 pmol/μl each	2 (1 μl each)
MgCl₂ (20 mM)	1 mM	1
dNTPs (2.5 mM each)	0.125 mM each	1
Taq polymerase (5 U/μl)	0.1 U/μl	0.4

(continued)

Reagent	Final concentration	Volume (μl)
ddH$_2$O		12.6 μl
Total volume		20 μl

5. Perform the PCR reaction using the below cycling conditions:

Initial incubation	95 °C	5 min
Denaturation	94 °C	30 s
Annealing	55–60 °C[a]	45 s
Extension	72 °C	45 s[a]
Final incubation	72 °C	3 min
Cycles	35	

[a]Depending on the oligonucleotides used, the annealing temperature and the extension time should be adjusted.

6. Analyze PCR products by gel electrophoresis. Load 5 μl of PCR products with loading dye onto 1% agarose gel (*see* Note **10**).

3.6 Tetrad Analysis (According to [15])

Tetrad analysis is performed to check whether the positive colonies screened by check PCR contain any extra mutations (*see* Note **11**).

1. Transform a heterozygous deletion mutant with pON177, a sporulation-inducing plasmid [16].

2. Allow the transformed cells to germinate for 3–4 days at 30 °C on minimal (+ adenine and leucine) plates.

3. Dissect the spores using a Singer MSM micromanipulator on YES plates at 25 °C and incubate the plates at 30 °C for 2–3 days.

4. Patch colonies onto YES plates and incubate at 30 °C for 3–4 days.

5. Re-patch viable colonies onto YES + 100 μg/ml G418 plates to confirm that viability is linked to G418 sensitivity. Correct deletion mutants are detected as G418-resistant colonies, while wild-type cells are not viable.

4   Notes

1. The *S. pombe* genome-wide deletion mutant library is commercially available from *Bioneer, Inc.*, 1301 Marina Village Pkwy, Suite 110, Alameda, CA 94501, USA. Phone: (510)

865-0330, Fax: (510) 865-0350. E-mail: order.usa@bioneer. us.com. Single-gene deletion strains can be obtained from the Yeast Genetic Resource Center at Osaka City University, Osaka, Japan.

2. The KanMX4 sequence is available at http://pombe.kaist. ac.kr/nbtsupp/protocols/KanMX4_GS.pdf.

3. The LCR is carried out using *Tfi* DNA ligase, which is purified from a recombinant *E. coli* strain encoding a *Thermus filiformis* DNA ligase. This enzyme is a thermo-stable DNA ligase whose stability and catalytic activity are well maintained under high temperature conditions (45–65 °C) compared to conventional DNA ligases, making it an ideal enzyme for high-temperature and high-stringency ligation. *Tfi* DNA ligase is available from:

   Bioneer, Inc., 1301 Marina Village Pkwy, Suite 110, Alameda, CA 94501, USA. Phone: (510) 865-0330, Fax: (510) 865-0350. E-mail: order.usa@bioneer.us.com.

4. There are many free software available for secondary structure prediction such as RNAfold Web Server (http://rna.tbi.univie. ac.at/cgi-bin/RNAfold.cgi) [18] and mFold Web Server (http://mfold.rna.albany.edu/?q=mfold/download-mfold) [19]. Barcode sequences can be checked for homology against genomic sequences using Basic Local Alignment Search Tool (BLAST, http://blast.ncbi.nlm.nih.gov/Blast.cgi). Details on the generation of the barcode region and artificial linker sequences are provided in [5].

5. The importance of determining an optimal ligation temperature is well demonstrated in exemplary experiments using deletion cassettes targeting *urm1* (ubiquitin family protein, SPCC548.04) and *srp14* (signal recognition particle subunit, SPAC19B12.09). The oligonucleotides for these two cassettes were ligated at three different temperatures, 54.3, 56.3, and 58.6 °C, and then the LCR products were subjected to the first round of nested PCR, which did not produce discrete visible bands on an agarose gel (Fig. 4a) [3]. The second round of nested PCR was carried out using different dilutions of the first-round nested PCR products, ranging from 20-fold (1 out of 20 µl) to 80-fold (0.25 out of 20 µl). As shown in Fig. 4b, the second-round nested PCR was successful for the LCR products ligated at 58.6 °C, irrespective of the degree of dilution, whereas the reactions with the LCR products ligated at 54.3 or 56.3 °C yielded no or incorrectly sized bands [3]. These results indicate that the success of deletion cassette amplification is critically dependent on the LCR performed at an optimal ligation temperature.

6. The artificial linkers could interrupt homologous recombination and should be removed to achieve a maximum success rate. It has been shown that the success rate for Eco31I-digested deletion cassettes increases by up to tenfold compared to undigested deletion cassettes [3].

7. Eco31I can be eliminated either by gel purification or by heat inactivation. It was demonstrated that there is little difference in resulting transformation yield (which is defined as number of colonies per 1 μg of deletion cassette) between the two methods [3].

8. The generation time of S. *pombe* is about 2–4 h at 30 °C, which can vary depending on strain background and culture medium. To ensure that log-phase cells are used, inoculate a few liquid cultures with different cell densities and incubate for 12 h [7].

9. It is critical to use cells in logarithmic growth phase for high transformation efficiency.
Log-phase cells are 7–14 μm long and have a cylindrical morphology with about 10–20% showing a septum [7].

10. If the deletion is not successful and no PCR product is generated, another round of PCR is performed using the cp5i and cp3i primers inside the CDS to confirm that the gene coding sequence is still present (Fig. 2b). After agarose gel electrophoresis, the PCR product from each successful deletion mutant is examined by dideoxy sequencing to confirm the sequences of up- and down-tags as well as across the junctions to accurately define the region deleted. All confirmed S. *pombe* deletion mutants are kept as 40% frozen glycerol stocks.

11. The results of tetrad analysis have been shown to be positive for check PCR-verified colonies [3], which suggests that check PCR is a highly reliable verification method.

References

1. Rothstein R (1991) Targeting, disruption, replacement, and allele rescue: integrative DNA transformation in yeast. Methods Enzymol 194:281–301

2. Johnston M, Riles L, Hegemann JH (2002) Gene disruption. Methods Enzymol 350:290–315

3. Nam M, Lee SJ, Han S et al (2014) Systematic targeted gene deletion using the gene-synthesis method in fission yeast. J Microbiol Methods 106:72–77. doi:10.1016/j.mimet.2014.08.005

4. Shoemaker DD, Lashkari DA, Morris D et al (1996) Quantitative phenotypic analysis of yeast deletion mutants using a highly parallel molecular bar-coding strategy. Nat Genet 14(4):450–456. doi:10.1038/ng1296-450

5. Kim DU, Hayles J, Kim D et al (2010) Analysis of a genome-wide set of gene deletions in the fission yeast Schizosaccharomyces pombe. Nat Biotechnol 28(6):617–623. doi:10.1038/nbt.1628

6. Giaever G, Chu AM, Ni L et al (2002) Functional profiling of the Saccharomyces cerevisiae genome. Nature 418(6896):387–391. doi:10.1038/nature00935

7. Hegemann JH, Heick SB, Pohlmann J et al (2014) Targeted gene deletion in Saccharomyces cerevisiae and Schizosaccharomyces pombe. Methods Mol Biol 1163:45–73. doi:10.1007/978-1-4939-0799-1_5

8. Hegemann JH, Heick SB (2011) Delete and repeat: a comprehensive toolkit for sequential gene knockout in the budding yeast Saccharomyces cerevisiae. Methods Mol Biol 765:189–206. doi:10.1007/978-1-61779-197-0_12

9. Winzeler EA, Shoemaker DD, Astromoff A et al (1999) Functional characterization of the S. cerevisiae genome by gene deletion and parallel analysis. Science 285(5429): 901–906

10. Decottignies A, Sanchez-Perez I, Nurse P (2003) Schizosaccharomyces pombe essential genes: a pilot study. Genome Res 13(3):399–406. doi:10.1101/gr.636103

11. Manivasakam P, Weber SC, McElver J et al (1995) Micro-homology mediated PCR targeting in Saccharomyces cerevisiae. Nucleic Acids Res 23(14):2799–2800

12. Rothstein RJ (1983) One-step gene disruption in yeast. Methods Enzymol 101:202–211

13. Bahler J, Wu JQ, Longtine MS et al (1998) Heterologous modules for efficient and versatile PCR-based gene targeting in Schizosaccharomyces pombe. Yeast 14(10):943–951. doi:10.1002/(SICI)1097-0061(199807)14:10<943::AID-YEA292>3.0.CO;2-Y

14. Gregan J, Rabitsch PK, Sakem B et al (2005) Novel genes required for meiotic chromosome segregation are identified by a high-throughput knockout screen in fission yeast. Curr Biol 15(18):1663–1669. doi:10.1016/j.cub.2005.07.059

15. Moreno S, Klar A, Nurse P (1991) Molecular genetic analysis of fission yeast Schizosaccharomyces pombe. Methods Enzymol 194:795–823

16. Styrkarsdottir U, Egel R, Nielsen O (1993) The smt-0 mutation which abolishes mating-type switching in fission yeast is a deletion. Curr Genet 23(2):184–186

17. SantaLucia J Jr (1998) A unified view of polymer, dumbbell, and oligonucleotide DNA nearest-neighbor thermodynamics. Proc Natl Acad Sci U S A 95(4):1460–1465

18. Gruber AR, Lorenz R, Bernhart SH et al (2008) The Vienna RNA websuite. Nucleic Acids Res 36(Web Server Issue):W70–W74. doi:10.1093/nar/gkn188

19. Zuker M (2003) Mfold web server for nucleic acid folding and hybridization prediction. Nucleic Acids Res 31(13):3406–3415

Chapter 14

Efficient Assembly of DNA Using Yeast Homologous Recombination (YHR)

Sunil Chandran and Elaine Shapland

Abstract

The assembly of multiple DNA parts into a larger DNA construct is a requirement in most synthetic biology laboratories. Here we describe a method for the efficient, high-throughput, assembly of DNA utilizing the yeast homologous recombination (YHR). The YHR method utilizes overlapping DNA parts that are assembled together by *Saccharomyces cerevisiae* via homologous recombination between designed overlapping regions. Using this method, we have successfully assembled up to 12 DNA parts in a single reaction.

Key words Synthetic biology, DNA assembly, High throughput, Yeast homologous recombination, DNA synthesis

1 Introduction

The assembly of DNA parts into larger DNA assemblies is a routine operation in most synthetic biology laboratories. DNA constructs, ranging in length from 3 to 20 kb and consisting of 2–12 DNA parts can be routinely assembled and introduced into strains for various applications. While numerous DNA assembly methods are currently available [1, 2], they are all limited in the number of DNA parts that can be assembled, or have inconvenient assembly methodologies, or are not amenable to high-throughput operations. As a host, *Saccharomyces cerevisiae* is unmatched in its ability to facilitate homologous recombination. This ability has been successfully co-opted by multiple groups to assemble large DNA plasmids with high efficiency [3]. The method relies on transforming DNA parts and a linearized shuttle vector with homologous ends into a yeast host (Fig. 1). Using homology lengths between 24 and 36 bp, we have managed to successfully assemble DNA constructs containing up to 12 DNA parts [4] (*see* **Note 1**)

Randall A. Hughes (ed.), *Synthetic DNA: Methods and Protocols*, Methods in Molecular Biology, vol. 1472,
DOI 10.1007/978-1-4939-6343-0_14, © Springer Science+Business Media New York 2017

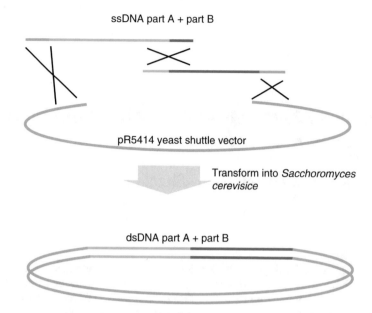

Fig. 1 Mechanism of assembly via yeast homologous recombination (YHR). Each DNA part is amplified with oligonucleotides that incorporate a small sequence from the adjacent DNA part, resulting in a homology of 24–36 bp between each adjacent DNA part. Transforming the parts into *S. cerevisiae* enables the DNA parts to be assembled into a plasmid

2   Materials

2.1   Reagents for DNA Part Amplification, Purification, and Assembly

1. Phusion Hot-Start Flex DNA Polymerase with supplied 10× buffer and dNTPs (New England Biolabs).

2. DpnI (New England Biolabs).

3. AxyPrep Mag PCR clean-up kit (Axygen Scientific) or similar.

4. XL1-Blue chemically competent *E. coli* cells.

5. pRS414 yeast shuttle vector (ATCC® 87519™).

6. *Saccharomyces cerevisiae* strain CEN.PK2-1c (*29, 30*), tryptophan auxotroph (*MATa ura3-52 trp1-289 leu2-3,112 his3Δ1 MAL2-8C SUC2*).

7. Zymoprep yeast plasmid miniprep kit (Zymo Research, Irvine, CA).

8. Commercially synthesized oligonucleotides.

9. 0.2 mL thin-walled PCR tubes.

10. 1.5 mL microcentrifuge tubes.

11. 50% PEG 3500 solution (95904 Sigma or similar).

12. Agarose gel: Agarose Molecular Biology Grade (Fisher part number BP1356-100). Place gel trays into the casting tray, place the comb of your choice into the slot in the gel tray. Add 1 g of agarose to a clean 250 mL bottle or flask. Add 100 mL 1× TAE Buffer. Microwave until dissolved. Allow to cool to approximately 65 °C. Add 5 μL ethidium bromide solution. Swirl, carefully, keeping bottle top or neck of flask pointed away from you. Pour. (100 mL ≈ two 7 cm × 10 cm gels.). After the gel has hardened, remove comb and store in 1× TAE bath, at room temperature, for up to 7 days.

13. 1× TE buffer: 10 mM Tris–HCl pH 8.0, 1 mM EDTA.

14. Salmon sperm DNA (ssDNA) 10 mg/L (Thermo Fisher 15632-011 or similar).

15. LB broth: Use LB Broth (powdered) (Fisher P/N BP1426 or similar). Add 900 mL of dH$_2$O to a clean 1 L flask or bottle. Add 25 g of LB broth to the flask or bottle. Stir until powder is dissolved. Transfer the solution to a 1 L graduated cylinder and add diH$_2$O until the total volume of 1 L is reached. Transfer the solution to a glass media bottle. Loosely cap and sterilize by autoclaving for 20 min at 15 psi (1.05 kg/cm^2) on liquid cycle.

16. YPD (1% yeast extract, 2% peptone, 2% dextrose): To a 2 L beaker add 10 g yeast extract (BD 211677 or similar) and 20 g peptone (BD 211929 or similar) and 700 mL of dH$_2$O and stir until powder is dissolved. Transfer the solution to a 1 L graduated cylinder and add DiH$_2$O until the total volume of 900 mL is reached. Transfer the solution to a glass media bottle. Loosely cap and sterilize by autoclaving for 20 min at 15 psi (1.05 kg/cm^2) on liquid cycle. Allow it to cool and add 100 mL of 20% glucose.

17. CSM-W (complete yeast synthetic medium without tryptophan): To a 2 L beaker add 700 mL of dH$_2$O and a stir bar. Add 0.74 g of CSM without tryptophan (114511012 MP BIOMEDICALS or similar) and 43.7 g DOB (114025012 MP BIOMEDICALS or similar) and stir until dissolved. Transfer the solution to a glass media bottle. Loosely cap and sterilize by autoclaving for 20 min at 15 psi (1.05 kg/cm^2) on liquid cycle.

2.2 Equipment

1. Thermocycler.

2. Fragment analyzer (optional).

3. Agarose gel electrophoresis equipment (gel rigs, casting trays, combs).

4. Bacterial cultivation equipment (shakers, incubators).

5. Spectrophotometer (NanoDrop or similar).

3   Methods

3.1   Design of Bridging Oligonucleotides

1. Design oligonucleotides for each DNA part (including the shuttle vector) to include 20–30 bp that anneal to that DNA part ($T_m \sim 60$ °C) and 24–36 bp that anneal to the adjacent DNA part (*see* **Note 2**).

2. Order desalted bridging oligonucleotides from commercial oligonucleotide supplier.

3.2   Preparation of DNA Parts for Assembly

1. Set up PCR reactions to amplify all of the component parts to perform the assembly as per the Phusion DNA polymerase supplier recommended conditions (https://www.neb.com/protocols/1/01/01/pcr-protocol-m0530). In general, in a 0.2 mL PCR tube add 10–100 ng of template DNA, 1× Phusion Hot-Start Flex buffer, 200 µM dNTP's, 0.5 µM Forward primer, 0.5 µM Reverse primer, 1 unit of Phusion Hot-Start Flex DNA polymerase and water to a final volume of 50 µL.

2. Amplify each DNA part using the conditions recommended by the Phusion DNA polymerase supplier (e.g., https://www.neb.com/protocols/1/01/01/pcr-protocol-m0530). Adjust the annealing and extension conditions specific to the primers and lengths specific to each DNA part. In general, use the following temperature cycles: 1 cycle of 30 s at 98 °C, 30 cycles of denaturation at 98 °C for 10 s; annealing for 30 s at a temperature specific to the primers T_m (preferably between 55 and 60 °C) and extension at 72 °C for a time period specific to the length of each DNA part (15–30 s extension time per kb of DNA); 1 cycle of 4 min at 72 °C; incubation at 4 °C till the samples are analyzed.

3. Verify the successful amplification of the component parts by running a 5 µL aliquot of each PCR on a 1% agarose gel. Visualize the gel on a transilluminator or gel imaging system.

4. In the case of the amplified shuttle vector as well as any DNA part that is amplified from plasmid DNA, treat with DpnI as follows to remove the plasmid DNA template. To a 50 µL PCR reaction generated above add 20 U DpnI followed by incubation for 60 min at 37 °C and 20 min at 65 °C to degrade the methylated plasmid DNA.

5. Purify the PCR amplified DNA parts using the AxyPrep Mag PCR clean-up kit (or similar PCR clean-up kit) according to manufacturer's instructions. Purify 150 µL worth of PCR reaction mixture and concentrate the sample by eluting into 45 µL 1× TE Buffer.

6. Analyze the DNA parts for the correct fragment size and purity using capillary electrophoresis on a fragment analyzer or by agarose gel electrophoresis. Measure the DNA concentrations using a spectrophotometer.

**3.3   DNA Assembly
via Yeast Homologous
Recombination**

1. Inoculate 5 mL YPD with a single yeast colony and incubate overnight in 30 °C with shaking.

2. Inoculate 25 mL YPD with overnight culture to an OD600 ~ 0.175–0.200.

3. Grow culture with shaking at 30 °C to an OD600 ~ 0.7–0.9 (3–5 h, sometimes longer). Alternatively, inoculate 25 mL YPD overnight culture directly with a very small amount of cells from a colony to achieve an OD600 ~ 0.7–0.9 the next morning.

4. Harvest 5 mL of culture in 15 mL conical tubes by spinning at max speed for 1 min.

5. Resuspend pellet in 5–10 mL of H_2O. Spin down for 1 min at max speed.

6. Remove supernatant and resuspend pellet in 1 mL H_2O and transfer to labeled microcentrifuge tube. Spin down at high speed for 30 s.

7. Remove supernatant and wash pellet in 1 mL 100 mM LiAc. Spin at high speed for 30 s.

8. Remove supernatant and add in the following in order:

   (a) 240 μL 50% PEG 3500 solution.

   (b) 36 μL 1.0 M LiAc.

   (c) 10 μL ssDNA (10 mg/mL) that has been previously boiled at 95 °C for 10 min and immediately placed on ice.

   (d) 21 μL DNA part mix containing 150 fmol of each DNA part and 5 fmol shuttle vector.

   (e) 54 μL ddH₂O.

9. Vortex for 30 s or until becomes a homogenous suspension.

10. Incubate the cells in a thermal cycler for 30 min at 30 °C, then heat-shock for 45 min at 42 °C, followed by incubation for 15–45 min at 25 °C.

11. After heat shock, wash the cells and resuspend in 1000 μL complete yeast synthetic medium without tryptophan.

12. Upon a 2-day outgrowth period (30 °C, with shaking), isolate the assembled plasmid DNA using the Zymoprep yeast plasmid miniprep II kit and elute in 40 μL 1× TE.

**3.4   Transformation
to E. coli, Colony
Counting,
and Restriction
Endonuclease DNA
Fragment Analysis**

1. Transform 10 μL of the yeast miniprep into 40 μL XL1-Blue chemically competent *E. coli* cells (3–5×10^7 CFUs/μg pUC19) according to manufacturer's instructions.

2. After transformation, dilute the cells in Luria broth (LB) and plate on LB agar plates containing 100 μg/mL carbenicillin.

3. After overnight incubation at 37 °C, count the colony forming units (CFUs). Pick colonies (up to 30 per assembly reaction, if available) into liquid LB medium containing 100 μg/mL carbenicillin.

4. Shake overnight at 37 °C and isolate the plasmids via standard miniprep protocols and analyze via sequencing or restriction digest analysis for the correct clone.

4 Notes

1. As with any assembly method, the efficiency of the YHR assembly method tends to drop as the number of DNA parts or the size of the entire construct increases. This method has been successfully utilized to assemble up to 12 DNA parts (0.5–2.5 kb each). The number of DNA parts can theoretically be increased with an increase in the homology size between DNA parts.

2. Amplification oligos should be 25–30 bp long and have a T_m of 60 °C for best results.

Acknowledgements

This work was funded by Defense Advanced Research Projects Agency (DARPA) Living Foundries grant HR001-12-3-0006.

References

1. Ellis T, Adie T, Baldwin GS (2011) DNA assembly for synthetic biology: from parts to pathways and beyond. Integr Biol 3:109–118

2. Merryman C, Gibson DG (2012) Methods and applications for assembling large DNA constructs. Metab Eng 14:196–204

3. Gibson DG, Benders GA, Axelrod KC, Zaveri J, Algire MA, Moodie M, Montague MG, Venter JC, Smith HO, Hutchison CA (2008) One-step assembly in yeast of 25 overlapping DNA fragments to form a complete synthetic *Mycoplasma genitalium* genome. Proc Natl Acad Sci U S A 105:20404–20409

4. de Kok S, Stanton LH, Slaby T, Durot M, Holmes VF, Patel KG, Platt D, Shapland EB, Serber Z, Dean J et al (2014) Rapid and reliable DNA assembly via ligase cycling reaction. ACS Synth Biol 3:97–106

Chapter 15

Simultaneous Removal of Multiple DNA Segments by Polymerase Chain Reactions

Vishnu Krishnamurthy and Kai Zhang

Abstract

Precise DNA manipulation is a key enabling technology for synthetic biology. Approaches based on restriction digestion are often limited by the presence of certain restriction enzyme recognition sites. Recent development of restriction-free cloning approaches has greatly enhanced the flexibility and speed of molecular cloning. Most restriction-free cloning methods focus on DNA assembly. Much less work has been dedicated towards DNA removal. Here we introduce a protocol that allows simultaneous removal of multiple DNA segments from a plasmid using polymerase chain reactions (PCR). Our approach will be beneficial to applications in multiple sites mutagenesis, DNA library construction, genetic and protein engineering, and synthetic biology.

Key words Restriction-free cloning, Polymerase chain reaction, Synthetic DNA assembly and manipulation, Multiplex gene removal, Synthetic single-stranded bridging oligos

1 Introduction

Synthetic biology is an emerging interdisciplinary branch of biology that spans biotechnology, biophysics, biochemistry, and engineering [1]. It aims to design and construct biological modules, devices, systems, networks, and machines to rewire and reprogram biological organisms [2]. A key enabling technology in synthetic biology is precise manipulation and assembly of synthetic DNA constructs. Conventional approaches of DNA manipulation depend on restriction enzyme digestion, followed by ligation. Such approaches are limited by the presence of unique, specific restriction enzyme recognition sites, which are not necessarily available in a plasmid. Consequently, site-directed mutagenesis of genes is often needed to insert appropriate digestion sites, the use of which can affect endogenous structure and function of the encoded protein.

Restriction-free DNA cloning technologies have successfully removed limitations in restriction enzyme-based methods [3]. DNA assembly can be achieved by end-homology recombination

Randall A. Hughes (ed.), *Synthetic DNA: Methods and Protocols*, Methods in Molecular Biology, vol. 1472,
DOI 10.1007/978-1-4939-6343-0_15, © Springer Science+Business Media New York 2017

methods including Gateway, overlap extension PCR [4], transfer PCR [5], DNA fragment assembly [6], restriction-free (RF) cloning [7], circular polymerase extension cloning (CPEC) [8], seamless ligation cloning extract (SLiCE) [9], and prolonged overlap extension PCR (POE-PCR) [10]. Alternative methods based on DNA annealing include ligation-independent cloning (LIC) [11], In-Fusion [12], quick and clean (QC) cloning [13], sequence and ligation-independent cloning (SLIC) [14], Gibson [15], ligase cycling reaction (LCR) [16, 17], and PaperClip [18]. Approaches for mutation include single primer mutagenesis (SOMA) [19], simultaneous noncontiguous deletion [20], and multiplexing clonality [21]. Most of these restriction-free cloning approaches primarily target DNA assembly or mutation. Much less work has been devoted to DNA removal. The ability to remove specific DNA sequences is critical for structure-function analysis of proteins, DNA library construction, as well as genetic and protein engineering.

Here we introduce a PCR-based restriction-free cloning technique that allows simultaneous removal of multiple DNA segments from a plasmid (Fig. 1) [22]. We demonstrate simultaneous three-gene removal from a plasmid pCRII-U85 in a one-pot reaction. By properly designing gene-specific primers, one would be able to apply the same protocol to remove any DNA segments from a plasmid. The pCRII-U85 plasmid has a *u85* gene inserted into the *lacZ* sequence within the pCRII vector, which has both kanamycin

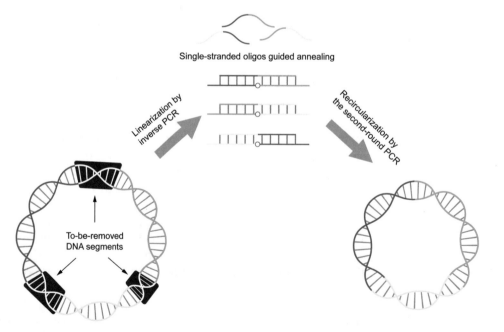

Fig. 1 Overall scheme of multiple gene removal based on two-step polymerase chain reactions. The first round of PCR generates linear products, which are recombined by the second round of PCR guided by complementary single-stranded oligos

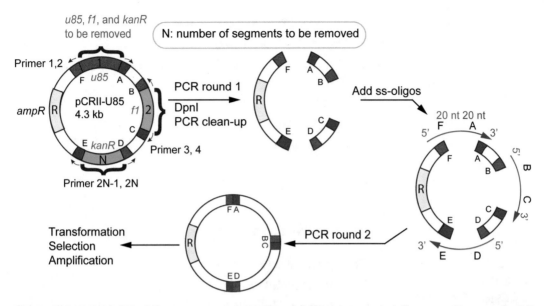

Fig. 2 pCRII-U85 plasmid with gene segments *u85*, *f1*, and *kanR* to be removed. To remove N segments, 2 N primers are used to generate N linear fragments in the first round of PCR. The product mixture is then treated with DpnI to remove the original template, followed by PCR clean-up. To set up the second round of PCR, fresh master mix and N ss-oligos are added to the purified PCR products. Each oligo shares a 20-nt complementarity to two neighboring fragments to be connected. Final PCR products containing nicked plasmids are used in transformation. Reproduced from [22] with permission from Elsevier

and ampicillin resistance genes (*kanR* and *ampR*). This construct allows quick readout of successful gene removal. We will simultaneously remove *u85*, *kanR*, and part of *f1-ori* (abbreviated as *f1*) segments from pCRII-U85 (Fig. 2). Removal of *u85* should produce blue colonies in a blue/white colony screening assay; removal of *kanR* while retaining *ampR* should allow colonies to grow selectively only on ampicillin plates. The final sequences are confirmed by DNA sequencing. By using synthetic single-stranded oligos as bridging sequences, our approach does not require alteration of template DNA to create overlap between neighboring segments. Consequently, this approach does not produce residual sequence between neighboring segments.

2   Materials

2.1   Components for Two-Step PCR Reaction

1. Oligonucleotides as primer pairs: 10 μM in Molecular grade water.

2. Guiding single-stranded oligonucleotides (ss-oligos): 20 μM in Molecular grade water.

3. Plasmid template: 10 pg/μL in Molecular grade water.

4. 2× Phusion DNA polymerase master mix.

5. 2× DreamTaq PCR master mix.

6. 1× TAE buffer: 40 mM Tris, 20 mM acetic acid, and 1 mM EDTA.

7. DNA ladder.

8. DpnI: 10 U/μL.

9. Agarose gel apparatus.

10. PCR clean-up kit.

11. Thermocycler.

12. Nanodrop.

13. Blue transilluminator.

2.2 Components for Confirmation of Successful Removal of DNA Segments

1. Competent cells (e.g., DH5α).

2. Luria-Bertani (LB) medium.

3. Luria-Bertani (LB) agar plate with appropriate antibiotics (e.g., ampicillin or kanamycin-resistant).

4. 5-Bromo-4-chloro-3-indolyl β-D-galactopyranoside (X-gal) stock solution: 20 mg/mL in dimethylformamide (DMF).

5. 14 mL sterile cell culture tubes.

6. Agarose gel premixed with SYBR green.

7. Agarose gel apparatus.

8. Minicentrifuge.

9. Shaker incubator.

3   Methods

3.1 Primer Design

1. For each gene segment to be removed, three nonphosphory-lated primers are designed: two for the first round of PCR and one for the second round of PCR.

2. For the first round of PCR, design primers so that the sense primer is the vector sequence downstream of the gene to be excised and the antisense primer is the reverse complement of the vector sequence upstream of the gene to be excised (Fig. 2).

3. Vary the length of both primers between 18 and 22 bases so that their annealing temperatures are within 4 °C of each other.

4. For the second round of PCR, design a 40-base single-stranded oligo with a 20-nt complementarity to each of the two fragments to be connected (Fig. 2).

**3.2   Linearization
by the First-Step PCR**

1. To linearize the vector in the first round of PCR, mix 10 µL Phusion polymerase 2× master mix with 1 µL each of the sense and antisense primers (10 µM), 1 µL template (10 pg/µL), and 7 µL of water (*see* **Note 1**).

2. In each reaction cycle, the reaction mixture is denatured at 98 °C for 15 s, annealed for 15 s (*see* **Note 2**), and extended at 72 °C (*see* **Note 3**). Mixing multiple pairs of primers does not degrade the quality of linear products compared to separate primer pairs (Fig. 3).

3. Repeat the cycle 25 times before a final extension of 10 min at 72 °C.

4. Hold the tubes at 4 °C if not used immediately.

5. The first step of PCR product was mixed with 2 µL DpnI (10 U/µL) and incubated at 37 °C for 1 h (*see* **Note 4**).

**3.3   Clean-Up
of the PCR Product**

1. Clean up PCR product following manufacturer's instructions (*see* **Note 5**).

2. The final concentration of the fragments is measured by NanoDrop (*see* **Note 6**).

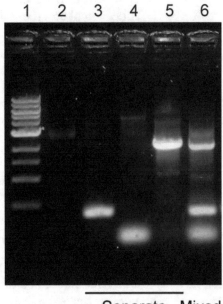

Fig. 3 Mixing three pairs of primers does not degrade the quality of linear products compared to separate primer pairs. *Lane 1*: DNA ladder, *Lane 2*: DNA template alone, *Lane 3–5*: PCR products with primer pair 1, 2, and 3 in three separate reactions, *Lane 6*: PCR products with all three pairs of primers mixed in one reaction. Reproduced from [23] with permission from Elsevier

3.4 Recircularization by the Second-Step PCR

1. Mix 250 ng of the PCR products (*see* **Note 7**) from the first round with 10 µL 2× Phusion polymerase master mix, 1 µL of ss-oligos (20 µM each, final concentration 1 µM), and water to make a 20 µL reaction mix.

2. In each reaction cycle, the reaction mixture is denatured at 98 °C for 15 s (*see* **Note 8**), annealed at 55 °C for 15 s, and extended at 72 °C (*see* **Note 9**). The reaction is repeated for 20 cycles.

3. The product is then ready for use in transformation. The transformation-ready product can be achieved within 8 h (PCR round 1: 2 h, DpnI treatment: 0.5 h, PCR clean-up 0.5 h, and PCR round 2: 3.5–4.5 h) (*see* **Note 10**).

3.5 Transformation and DNA Amplification

1. Thaw competent cells on ice for 10 min.

2. For each transformation reaction, transfer 30 µL competent cells to a sterile 14-mL culture tube. Incubate with 5 µL products of the second-round PCR on ice for 30 min (*see* **Note 11**).

3. Incubate the culture tube in a 42 °C water bath for exactly 45 s.

4. Transfer the culture tube back to ice and incubate for another 2 min.

5. Add 1 mL LB medium without antibiotics to the culture tube. Incubate the tube at 37 °C with vigorous shaking (225–250 rpm) for 1 h.

6. Spread 250 µL of cell culture evenly onto agar plates and incubate at 37 °C overnight.

3.6 Confirmation of Successful Removal of DNA Segments by Blue/White Colony Screen Assay

1. Spread 120 µL X-gal stock solution (20 mg/mL) to pre-made LB agar plates using a glass spreader at room temperature (*see* **Note 12**).

2. Incubate the plates at 37 °C for at least 30 min to dry.

3. Spread recovered competent cells onto the plates and incubate the plate at 37 °C overnight.

4. Colonies containing plasmids with successful DNA removal should appear blue (Fig. 4).

3.7 Confirmation of Successful Removal of DNA Segments by Colony PCR Reactions

1. For each colony to be tested, add 4 mL LB medium into a 14-mL sterile cell culture tube.

2. Use a sterile toothpick or pipette tip, pick a single colony from the agar plate.

3. Drop the tip or toothpick into the LB medium with appropriate antibiotics.

4. Repeat **steps 2–3** and randomly pick a total of 6–8 colonies from the same agar plate.

5. Incubate the cells at 37 °C for 4 h with vigorous shaking (*see* **Note 13**).

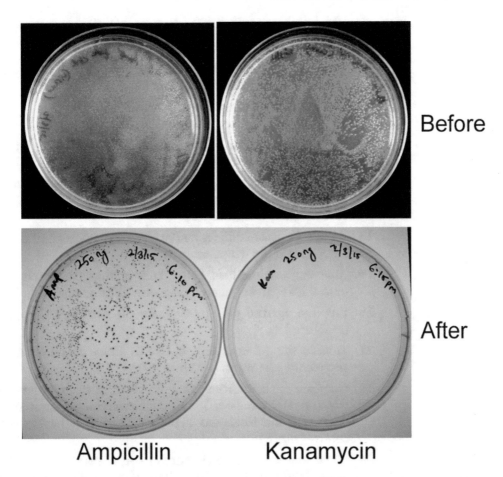

Fig. 4 Images of agar plates with plasmids before and after gene removal. Before gene removal, white colonies on ampicillin and kanamycin plates indicate that *u85*, *ampR*, and *kanR* genes were intact. After gene removal, *blue* colonies on the ampicillin plate indicate that *u85* was removed and *ampR* is intact; no colonies on the kanamycin plate indicate that *kanR* was removed. Reproduced from [22] with permission from Elsevier

6. Transfer 1 mL of cell culture to a 1.5 mL microcentrifuge tube (*see* **Note 14**).

7. Return the rest of the cell culture back to the shaker incubator (*see* **Note 15**).

8. Spin the cultures down at 13,000 rpm (15,700 rcf) for 1 min in a minicentrifuge (*see* **Note 16**).

9. Carefully remove the supernatant by decanting or with a pipette.

10. Resuspend each cell pellet with 50 μL sterile water with a pipette.

11. Place each tube into a 100 °C dry heat bath for 5 min to lyse the cells (*see* **Note 17**).

12. After cell lysis, transfer each tube to ice and incubate for 2 min.

13. Spin down the cell lysates at 13,000 rpm (15,700 rcf) for 1 min in a microcentrifuge.

14. Use 2 μL clear supernatants as the template for the following colony PCR reaction.

15. Use a full-length plasmid as a control.

16. For each reaction, mix 10 μL 2× DreamTaq master mix with 1 μL of sense and antisense primers (10 μM stock), 2 μL template, and 6 μL of water.

17. In each reaction cycle, the reaction mixture is denatured at 95 °C for 30 s, annealed for 30 s, and extended at 72 °C (1.5 min/kb) (*see* **Note 18**).

18. Repeat the cycle 20 times before a final extension of 10 min at 72 °C. Hold the temperature at 4 °C.

19. After the reaction, load 10 μL PCR product from each tube onto a 1% agarose gel premixed with SYBR green.

20. Run the agarose gel at 90 V for 30 min in TAE buffer (*see* **Note 19**).

21. Transfer the gel from the gel tray to a blue transilluminator and record gel images (*see* **Note 20**).

22. Compare the band from colony PCR with that from the control (no DNA removal). With DNA segments successfully removed, those bands should migrate faster than that from the control (Fig. 5).

23. For colonies that generate correct size of band, purify DNA using the rest of 3 mL culture 24 h after initial inoculation.

24. Confirm successful DNA removal by DNA sequencing.

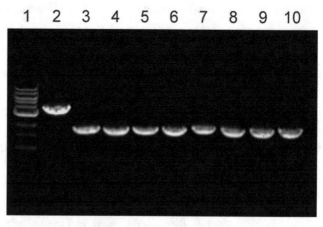

Fig. 5 Colony PCR showed that products from eight randomly selected colonies have all three gene segments (*u85*, *f1*, and *kanR*) removed from the plasmid pCRII-U85. *Lane 1*: DNA ladder, *Lane 2*: products of full-length pCRII-U85. *Lane 3–10*: products of eight randomly selected colonies. Reproduced from [23] with permission from Elsevier

4 Notes

1. Typically 1 pg to 5 ng template produces similar yield of PCR products. The amount of template should be adjusted so that residual template generates no false-positive colonies after transformation.

2. Use the Tm calculator for Phusion polymerase (e.g., from NEB website) to estimate the annealing temperature. When multiple primer pairs are used, use the lowest annealing temperature of all primers.

3. Given a processive rate of 1 kb/min for the polymerase, the extension time depends on the longest linear product (e.g., 2 min for a 2 kb linear product).

4. No buffer exchange is required for DpnI treatment.

5. PCR clean-up removes digested DNA template segments, primers, and enzymes. Use Molecular grade water to elute the PCR products.

6. A typical concentration of the products ranges from 30 to 50 ng/µL with 50 µL elution buffer.

7. The 250 ng products include a mixture of all three linear DNA segments from the PCR clean-up.

8. Longer denaturing time may degrade performance of Phusion polymerase.

9. The extension time depends on the longest DNA segments with 1 kb/min extension rate.

10. Fresh samples generate best results in transformation. Alternatively, intermediate products can be stored in a –20 °C freezer overnight to allow flexibility in schedule.

11. Extensive exposure of the competent cells to room temperature before heat shock can lead to loss of competency.

12. If the blue/white screen is preferred, select strains with *lacZ(del)M15* genotype that encodes a mutant form of β-galactosidase (also referred to as ω-peptide). Successful removal of the DNA segments from within the *LacZα* regenerates LacZα, which should rescue the activity of β-galactosidase via α-complementation. Other methods (e.g., colony PCR) can be used in more general cases of DNA removal.

13. Loosely cover the culture with a cap to ensure sufficient air flow.

14. A slightly turbid culture should appear if cells in the selected colony were successfully transformed.

15. These cell cultures will be used for DNA amplification for selected colonies 24 h after inoculation.

16. A cell pellet of about 1 mm² should appear at the bottom of the microcentrifuge tube.

17. Wear appropriate personal protective equipment (PPE) (safety goggle, mask etc.) as caps from the heated microcentrifuge tube may pop up. Alternatively, use microcentrifuge tubes with security lock.

18. An extension rate of 1.5 min/kb ensures complete extension reactions for DreamTaq polymerase.

19. A voltage setting of 5–8 V/cm is recommended.

20. Record the gel image immediately after gel electrophoresis. Leaving the gel in TAE buffer for extensive time may lead to broadening of DNA bands due to diffusion.

Acknowledgements

K.Z. thanks the funding support from the University of Illinois at Urbana-Champaign (UIUC).

References

1. Purnick PEM, Weiss R (2009) The second wave of synthetic biology: from modules to systems. Nat Rev Mol Cell Biol 10(6):410–422. doi:10.1038/nrm2698

2. Khalil AS, Collins JJ (2010) Synthetic biology: applications come of age. Nat Rev Genet 11(5):367–379. doi:10.1038/nrg2775

3. Lale R, Valla S (2014) DNA cloning and assembly methods. Springer, New York, NY. doi:10.1007/978-1-62703-764-8

4. Bryksin AV, Matsumura I (2010) Overlap extension PCR cloning: a simple and reliable way to create recombinant plasmids. Biotechniques 48(6):463–465. doi:10.2144/000113418

5. Erijman A, Dantes A, Bernheim R, Shifman JM, Peleg Y (2011) Transfer-PCR (TPCR): a highway for DNA cloning and protein engineering. J Struct Biol 175(2):171–177. doi:10.1016/j.jsb.2011.04.005

6. Zuo PJ, Rabie ABM (2010) One-step DNA fragment assembly and circularization for gene cloning. Curr Issues Mol Biol 12:11–16

7. van den Ent F, Lowe J (2006) RF cloning: a restriction-free method for inserting target genes into plasmids. J Biochem Biophys Methods 67(1):67–74. doi:10.1016/j.jbbm.2005.12.008

8. Quan JY, Tian JD (2009) Circular polymerase extension cloning of complex gene libraries and pathways. PLoS One 4(7):6441. doi:10.1371/Journal.Pone.0006441

9. Zhang Y, Werling U, Edelmann W (2012) SLiCE: a novel bacterial cell extract-based DNA cloning method. Nucleic Acids Res 40(8), e55. doi:10.1093/nar/gkr1288

10. You C, Zhang XZ, Zhang YH (2012) Simple cloning via direct transformation of PCR product (DNA Multimer) to Escherichia coli and Bacillus subtilis. Appl Environ Microbiol 78(5):1593–1595. doi:10.1128/AEM.07105-11

11. Aslanidis C, Dejong PJ (1990) Ligation-independent cloning of PCR products (LIC-PCR). Nucleic Acids Res 18(20):6069–6074. doi:10.1093/nar/18.20.6069

12. Raman M, Martin K (2014) One solution for cloning and mutagenesis: in-fusion (R) HD cloning plus. Nat Methods 11(9):Iii–V

13. Thieme F, Engler C, Kandzia R, Marillonnet S (2011) Quick and clean cloning: a ligation-independent cloning strategy for selective cloning of specific PCR products from non-specific mixes. PLoS One 6(6):12. doi:10.1371/journal.pone.0020556

14. Li MZ, Elledge SJ (2007) Harnessing homologous recombination in vitro to generate recombinant DNA via SLIC. Nat Methods 4(3):251–256. doi:10.1038/nmeth1010

15. Gibson DG, Young L, Chuang RY, Venter JC, Hutchison CA, Smith HO (2009) Enzymatic assembly of DNA molecules up to several hundred kilobases. Nat Methods 6(5):343–345. doi:10.1038/Nmeth.1318

16. de Kok S, Stanton LH, Slaby T, Durot M, Holmes VF, Patel KG, Platt D, Shapland EB, Serber Z, Dean J, Newman JD, Chandran SS (2014) Rapid and reliable DNA assembly via ligase cycling reaction. ACS Synth Biol 3(2):97–106. doi:10.1021/sb4001992

17. Paetzold B, Carolis C, Ferrar T, Serrano L, Lluch-Senar M (2013) In situ overlap and sequence synthesis during DNA assembly. ACS Synth Biol 2(12):750–755. doi:10.1021/sb400067v

18. Trubitsyna M, Michlewski G, Cai Y, Elfick A, French CE (2014) PaperClip: rapid multi-part DNA assembly from existing libraries. Nucleic Acids Res. doi:10.1093/nar/gku829

19. Pfirrmann T, Lokapally A, Andreasson C, Ljungdahl P, Hollemann T (2013) SOMA: a single oligonucleotide mutagenesis and cloning approach. PLoS One 8(6), e64870. doi:10.1371/journal.pone.0064870

20. Krishnakumar R, Grose C, Haft DH, Zaveri J, Alperovich N, Gibson DG, Merryman C, Glass JI (2014) Simultaneous non-contiguous deletions using large synthetic DNA and site-specific recombinases. Nucleic Acids Res 42(14), e111. doi:10.1093/nar/gku509

21. Cornils K, Thielecke L, Huser S, Forgber M, Thomaschewski M, Kleist N, Hussein K, Riecken K, Volz T, Gerdes S, Glauche I, Dahl A, Dandri M, Roeder I, Fehse B (2014) Multiplexing clonality: combining RGB marking and genetic barcoding. Nucleic Acids Res 42(7), e56. doi:10.1093/nar/gku081

22. Krishnamurthy VV, Khamo JS, Cho E, Schornak C, Zhang K (2015) Multiplex gene removal by two-step polymerase chain reactions. Anal Biochem 481:7–9. doi:10.1016/j.ab.2015.03.033

23. Krishnamurthy VV, Khamo JS, Cho E, Schornak C, Zhang K (2015) Polymerase chain reaction-based gene removal from plasmids. Data in Brief 4:75–82. doi:10.1016/j.dib.2015.04.024

Chapter 16

Rapid Construction of Recombinant Plasmids by QuickStep-Cloning

Pawel Jajesniak and Tuck Seng Wong

Abstract

QuickStep-Cloning is a novel molecular cloning technique that builds upon the concepts of asymmetric PCR and megaprimer-based amplification of whole plasmid. It was designed specifically to address the major drawbacks of previously reported cloning methods. The fully optimized protocol allows for a seamless integration of a long DNA fragment into any position within a plasmid of choice, in a time-efficient and cost-effective manner, without the need of a tedious DNA gel purification, a restriction digestion, and an enzymatic ligation. QuickStep-Cloning can be completed in less than 6 h, significantly faster than most of the existing cloning methods, while retaining high efficiency.

Key words Recombinant DNA, Megaprimer PCR, Ligation-independent cloning, Plasmid construction, Synthetic biology, Protein engineering, Metabolic engineering

1 Introduction

DNA cloning is, undoubtedly, one of the most fundamental molecular biology techniques. It is routinely employed in various disciplines related to genetic manipulation and is central to synthetic biology experiments. Conventionally, molecular cloning has been achieved by conducting a restriction enzyme digestion, followed by an enzymatic ligation. This approach, despite receiving unceasing support from the scientific community, is a resource-intensive procedure that depends on the availability of unique restriction sites and, potentially, results in addition of undesired amino acid(s). To address these problems, many sequence-independent cloning methods have been proposed in recent years [1]. Among these techniques, megaprimer-based cloning methods, such as restriction-free (RF) cloning [2] and MEGAWHOP cloning [3], are most popular for their simplicity and robustness. However, most megaprimer-based cloning methods rely on linear amplification of whole plasmid and the use of self-annealing megaprimers, which compromise their overall efficiency and significantly hinder their widespread adoption.

Randall A. Hughes (ed.), *Synthetic DNA: Methods and Protocols*, Methods in Molecular Biology, vol. 1472, DOI 10.1007/978-1-4939-6343-0_16, © Springer Science+Business Media New York 2017

QuickStep-Cloning utilizes asymmetric PCR to overcome the problem of self-annealing megaprimers and enables exponential amplification of recombinant plasmids [4]. QuickStep-Cloning consists of five simple steps (Fig. 1). The method begins with two parallel asymmetric PCRs. In each of these PCRs, DNA fragment of interest is amplified by two primers of unbalanced concentrations (1:50 ratio is used), resulting in predominantly single-stranded DNAs. Primers are designed in such a way that these single-stranded products carry a 3′-terminal region that corresponds to the integration site on the recipient plasmid. The two PCR mixtures are then purified separately. When mixed in an equimolar ratio, for the next PCR stage, the single-stranded products of the two asymmetric PCRs form megaprimer pairs, with 3′-overhangs that are complementary to the recipient plasmid. This allows megaprimers to anneal

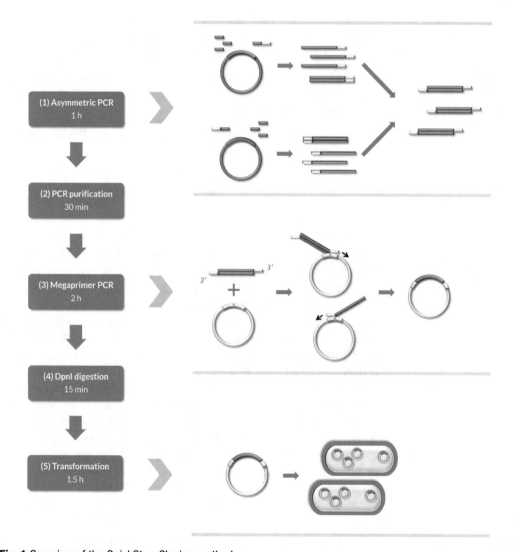

Fig. 1 Overview of the QuickStep-Cloning method

to the recipient plasmids, even when the two megaprimer strands self-anneal. Such a primer design also facilitates exponential amplification of whole plasmid [4], which results in the production of nicked-circular plasmids, with DNA fragment of interest integrated at the desired position. After a brief DpnI digestion to remove methylated/hemi-methylated parental plasmid, the PCR mixture is then used directly for bacterial transformation and protein expression. For a standard experiment involving cloning of a 1-kb DNA fragment into a 7-kb recipient plasmid, the aforementioned procedure can be completed in less than 6 h, without the need of lengthy enzymatic reactions or DNA gel purification [4]. Overall, QuickStep-Cloning is a robust method of constructing recombinant plasmids in a sequence-independent manner, with a reported cloning efficiency of over 90% [4].

2   Materials

2.1   Bacterial Strains

1. Competent *E. coli* cells (*see* **Note 1**).

2.2   Nucleic Acid

1. Donor plasmid (or other source of DNA insert; *see* **Note 2**).
2. Recipient plasmid.
3. PCR primers—*see* Subheading 3.1 for detailed information on primer design.

2.3   PCR Components

1. Q5 High-Fidelity DNA Polymerase (New England Biolabs, *see* **Note 3**).
2. Q5 Reaction Buffer (New England Biolabs).
3. Deoxynucleotide (dNTP) Solution Mix (New England Biolabs).
4. Ultrapure water.
5. 0.2 ml PCR tubes.
6. Thermal cycler (Eppendorf Mastercycler personal, or similar).

2.4   DpnI Digestion and DNA Purification

1. DpnI (New England Biolabs).
2. QIAquick PCR Purification Kit (Qiagen) or equivalent (*see* **Note 4**).
3. 1.5 or 2 ml microcentrifuge tubes.
4. Benchtop centrifuge (MiniSpin plus, or similar).
5. *Optional* Spectrophotometer.

2.5   Transformation and Clone Analysis

1. Ice.
2. 2×TY media: 16 g/L tryptone, 10 g/L yeast extract, and 5 g/L NaCl.

3. Agar plates supplemented with an appropriate antibiotic, e.g., TYE agar plates: 10 g/L tryptone, 5 g/L yeast extract, 8 g/L NaCl, and 15 g/L agar.

4. Sterile toothpicks.

5. 1.5 ml microcentrifuge tubes.

6. 50 ml sterile conical tubes.

7. QIAprep Spin Miniprep Kit (Qiagen) or equivalent.

8. Heat block (Eppendorf ThermoMixer C, or similar) or water bath.

9. Shaking incubator.

10. Incubator.

3 Methods

3.1 Primer Design

1. Identify DNA fragment to be cloned.

2. Using standard primer design guidelines, design a pair of oligonucleotides for amplification of the DNA fragment of interest (denoted herein as *Fwd* primer and *Rev* primer). Make sure that there is no significant difference between the melting temperatures of the two oligonucleotides (*see* **Note 5**).

3. Choose a DNA insertion point on the recipient plasmid.

4. Identify two megaprimer annealing sites (about 25 bp long) on both sides of the DNA insertion point and denote them as A and B (Fig. 2).

5. Check the melting temperatures (T_m) of both regions and adjust their length to obtain comparable melting temperatures (*see* **Note 5**).

6. Design primers *IntA-Fwd* and *IntB-Rev* according to Fig. 2. Remember to provide primer sequences in $5' \rightarrow 3'$ direction when placing the primer order.

3.2 Asymmetric PCR

1. Create 100 μM stock solutions of *Fwd*, *Rev*, *IntA-Fwd*, and *IntB-Rev* primers by resuspending the lyophilized oligonucleotides in ultrapure water (*see* **Note 6**). By diluting the 100 μM stock solution with ultrapure water, prepare 10 μM working solutions of *Fwd* and *Rev* primers and 0.2 μM working solutions of *IntA-Fwd* and *IntB-Rev* primers.

2. Prepare asymmetric PCR mixtures I and II (*see* Tables 1 and 2) in two separate 0.2 ml PCR tubes. Both mixtures should be prepared concurrently.

3. Transfer the two PCR tubes to a thermal cycler (*see* **Notes 7** and **8**) and initiate the thermocycling program given in Table 3.

4. Purify the two PCR products using QIAquick PCR Purification Kit (*see* **Note 4**). Elute with 30 μl of ultrapure water.

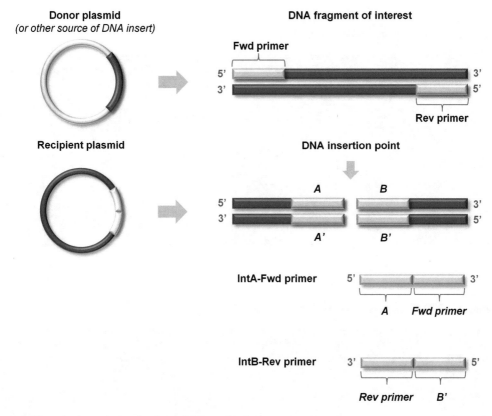

Fig. 2 Outline of primer design for the QuickStep-Cloning

Table 1
Composition of asymmetric PCR mixture I (*see* Note 2)

Component	Stock solution	Volume (μl)	Final concentration
Q5 Reaction Buffer	5×	10	1×
dNTP mix	10 mM each	1	0.2 mM each
Fwd primer	10 μM	2.5	0.5 μM
IntB-Rev primer	0.2 μM	2.5	0.01 μM
Donor plasmid	Variable	Variable	4 pg/μl
Q5 Polymerase	2 U/μl	0.5	0.02 U/μl
Ultrapure water		To 50 μl	

5. Quantify the DNA concentrations of the two purified products using a spectrophotometer (*see* **Note 9**). If no product is detected, consult **Note 10**.

6. Product of asymmetric PCR can be stored overnight at 4°C (if longer storage is required, place in −20°C freezer).

Table 2
Composition of asymmetric PCR mixture II (see Note 2)

Component	Stock solution	Volume (µl)	Final concentration
Q5 Reaction Buffer	5×	10	1×
dNTP mix	10 mM each	1	0.2 mM each
IntA-Fwd primer	0.2 µM	2.5	0.01 µM
Rev primer	10 µM	2.5	0.5 µM
Donor plasmid	Variable	Variable	4 pg/µl
Q5 Polymerase	2 U/µl	0.5	0.02 U/µl
Ultrapure water		To 50 µl	

Table 3
Asymmetric PCR thermocycling conditions (see Note 7)

Step	Temperature (°C)	Time	Cycles
Denaturation	98	30 s	1
Denaturation	98	7 s	30
Annealing	50–72	20 s	30
Elongation	72	30 s/kb	30
Cooling	4–8	–	–

3.3 Megaprimer PCR

1. Prepare megaprimer PCR mixture (**Table 4**) in a 0.2 ml PCR tube.

2. Transfer the PCR tube to a thermal cycler (*see* **Note 8**) and initiate the thermocycling program given in **Table 5** (*see* **Note 13**).

3. After the completion of PCR, add 2 µl of 20 U/µl DpnI directly into the 50 µl PCR product and incubate at 37 °C for 15 min (*see* **Note 14**).

4. For short-term storage, DpnI-digested PCR product can be kept at 4 °C. If longer storage is required, place in –20 °C freezer.

3.4 Transformation

1. Add 5 µl of the DpnI-treated reaction mixture (*see* **Note 15**) to 50–100 µl competent *E. coli* cells. Mix gently.

2. Incubate on ice for 30–60 min. Perform heat shock by placing the tube at 42 °C for 1 min. After the heat shock, transfer the tube immediately to ice for an additional 3 min incubation.

Table 4
Composition of megaprimer PCR mixture (*see* Note 11)

Component	Stock solution	Volume (µl)	Final concentration
Q5 Reaction Buffer	5×	10	1×
dNTP mix	10 mM each	1	0.2 mM each
Purified product of asymmetric PCR I	Variable	Variable	4 ng/µl
Purified product of asymmetric PCR II	Variable	Variable	4 ng/µl
Recipient plasmid	Variable	Variable	0.4 ng/µl
Q5 Polymerase	2 U/µl	0.5	0.02 U/µl
Ultrapure water		To 50 µl	

Table 5
Megaprimer PCR thermocycling conditions (*see* Note 12)

Step	Temperature (°C)	Time	Cycles
Denaturation	98	30 s	1
Denaturation	98	10 s	25
Annealing	50–72	20 s	25
Elongation	72	30 s/kb	25
Elongation	72	2 min	1
Cooling	4–8	–	–

3. Add 1 mL of 2×TY media (prewarmed to 37 °C) and incubate with shaking for 1 h at 37 °C.

4. Plate transformed cells on TYE agar plates supplemented with an appropriate antibiotic. Incubate overnight at 37 °C.

3.5 Colony Analysis

1. Inspect the plate for the presence of colonies (if no colonies are observed, consult **Note 16**).

2. Inoculate three colonies in separate 50 ml conical tubes containing 5 ml 2× TY media supplemented with an appropriate antibiotic. Incubate overnight at 37 °C with shaking.

3. Isolate the plasmids using QIAprep Spin Miniprep Kit.

4. Send the three plasmid samples for DNA sequencing to verify the presence of an insert at the desired position.

4   Notes

1. To prepare competent cells, traditional $CaCl_2$-based method was used [5]. It was found that, in QuickStep-Cloning, direct transformation of *E. coli* expression strain C41 (DE3) results in a higher number of transformants in comparison to transformation of DH5α cells. Competent cells prepared via more complicated protocols or purchased directly from a manufacturer (e.g., New England Biolabs) are fully compatible with the QuickStep-Cloning method and, more often than not, will result in a higher number of transformants. The use of commercially available ultracompetent cells is encouraged when attempting more challenging cloning experiments (e.g., in the case of cloning very long DNA fragments).

2. Sources of DNA insert other than a plasmid, e.g., a linear DNA fragment, can be used. However, it should be noted that the recommended DNA concentration, given in Tables 1 and 2, has been optimized for use with a 4-kb plasmid carrying a 1-kb DNA fragment of interest. When DNA fragments of significantly different molecular mass are to be used in the reaction, DNA concentration should be recalculated accordingly (knowing that the concentration given corresponds to 0.1 fmol molecules of cloned DNA fragment present in a 50 μl PCR mixture). When cloning very long DNA fragments (or other challenging amplicons), consult **Note 16**.

3. The protocol given has been carefully optimized for use with Q5 High-Fidelity DNA Polymerase from New England Biolabs; consequently, its use is strongly recommended. Other high-fidelity polymerases are, in principle, compatible with the concept of QuickStep-Cloning; however, their use necessitates a careful adjustment of the PCR conditions.

4. Other kits and alternative PCR purification methods can be used.

5. New England Biolabs provides a T_m calculator on its website, the use of which is strongly recommended.

6. When reconstituting the primers and preparing the oligonucleotide working solutions, TE buffer (10 mM Tris–HCl, 1 mM EDTA, pH 8.0) can be used instead of ultrapure water.

7. The annealing temperature should be calculated based on the sequence of *Fwd* and *Rev* primers (remember that only parts of *IntA-Fwd* and *IntB-Rev* primers anneal to the amplified DNA). Use of the New England Biolabs Tm Calculator is strongly recommended for this purpose. Time of the elongation step should be determined based on the length of the cloned DNA fragment (and not the length of a donor plasmid).

8. The two reaction mixtures should be transferred to a thermal cycler (preheated to 98 °C) immediately after their preparation.

9. Measuring DNA concentration at this point is strongly recommended as it helps to detect any potential problems with asymmetric PCRs and make sure that the amount of both megaprimers is sufficient for the second PCR stage. However, if the DNA quantification cannot be performed or is highly undesirable (e.g., in high-throughput applications), this step can be omitted.

10. Make sure that the primers have been correctly designed. The yield of asymmetric PCRs can be potentially improved by using a lower annealing temperature and a higher concentration of the donor plasmid (*see* **Note 14**).

11. The megaprimer concentrations, given in Table 4, have been optimized for use with a 1-kb insert. For longer inserts, use higher amounts of the megaprimer. If the two concentrations have not been measured or the yield of asymmetric PCR is insufficient to achieve the concentration given, use as high concentration as possible (i.e., if 1 μl of recipient plasmid is used, use 18.75 μl of purified asymmetric PCR product I and 18.75 μl of purified asymmetric PCR product II). The recipient plasmid concentration has been optimized for use with a 7-kb plasmid. If a recipient plasmid of significantly different molecular mass is used, recalculate the concentration accordingly.

12. The annealing temperature should be calculated based on the sequence of the two megaprimer annealing sites (denoted as A and B in Fig. 2). Use of the New England Biolabs Tm Calculator is strongly recommended for this purpose. The time of elongation step should be determined based on the total length of the recipient plasmid.

13. Higher yields of megaprimer PCR can be achieved by separating the two megaprimers for the first five PCR cycles. Two reaction mixtures (25 μl each; containing 1× Q5 Reaction Buffer, 200 μM of each dNTP, 200 ng of either purified asymmetric PCR product I or II, 10 ng of recipient plasmid, and 0.5 U Q5 High-Fidelity DNA Polymerase) are subjected to the thermocycling conditions of megaprimer PCR described in Table 5. After five cycles, they are mixed together and subjected to the remaining 20 cycles of the PCR program. This method is particularly useful in instances where low product yields are anticipated (e.g., in the case of cloning very long DNA fragments).

14. When using concentrations of donor or recipient plasmid that are significantly higher than the ones given in the protocol, it is recommended to increase DpnI digestion to 1 h to make sure all parental plasmids are properly digested.

15. As the transformation efficiency for intact cloning vectors is significantly higher than that for nicked plasmids, subjecting the product of megaprimer PCR to enzymatic phosphorylation and ligation can potentially increase the overall number of transformants.

16. The QuickStep-Cloning protocol has been optimized with the purpose of obtaining a significant number of transformants in the shortest time possible (at the same time, making sure that a high percentage of colonies contain a recombinant plasmid of interest). As a result, there are several simple strategies of modifying the protocol to increase the total number of transformants (in return for a more time-consuming procedure) that can be easily incorporated whenever the standard protocol does not provide desirable results (*see* **Notes 13** and **15**). Moreover, the yield of megaprimer PCR, and consequently the final number of transformants, can potentially be improved by using a lower annealing temperature, a higher concentration of the megaprimer, and/or a higher concentration of the recipient plasmid (*see* **Note 14**). Use of ultracompetent cells might also prove helpful (*see* **Note 1**).

References

1. Tee KL, Wong TS (2013) Polishing the craft of genetic diversity creation in directed evolution. Biotechnol Adv 31:1707–1721

2. van den Ent F, Lowe J (2006) RF cloning: a restriction-free method for inserting target genes into plasmids. J Biochem Biophys Methods 67:67–74

3. Miyazaki K (2011) MEGAWHOP cloning: a method of creating random mutagenesis libraries via megaprimer PCR of whole plasmids. Methods Enzymol 498:399–406

4. Jajesniak P, Wong TS (2015) QuickStep-Cloning: a sequence-independent, ligation-free method for rapid construction of recombinant plasmids. J Biol Eng 9:15

5. Hanahan D (1983) Studies on transformation of Escherichia coli with plasmids. J Mol Biol 166:557–580

Part III

Reducing Error in Synthetic DNA

Chapter 17

Immobilized MutS-Mediated Error Removal of Microchip-Synthesized DNA

Wen Wan, Dongmei Wang, Xiaolian Gao, and Jiong Hong

Abstract

Applications of microchip-synthesized oligonucleotides for de novo gene synthesis are limited primarily by their high error rates. The mismatch binding protein MutS, which can specifically recognize and bind to mismatches, is one of the cheapest tools for error correction of synthetic DNA. Here, we describe a protocol for removing errors in microchip-synthesized oligonucleotides and for the assembly of DNA segments using these oligonucleotides. This protocol can also be used in traditional de novo gene DNA synthesis.

Key words MutS, Microchip-synthesized oligonucleotides, Gene assemble, Error removal, De novo gene synthesis

1 Introduction

De novo gene synthesis is playing an increasingly important role in synthetic biology, systems biology, and general biomedical sciences [1–4]. De novo gene synthesis relies on the chemical synthesis of oligonucleotides (oligos) to supply building blocks for enzymatic assembly [5, 6]. Compared to typically used controlled-pore glass-synthesized oligos (CPG-oligos), microchip-synthesized oligos (Mcp-oligos) are advantageous due to the high oligo synthesis throughput (10^3–10^6 oligos per chip) and low synthesis cost ($0.00001–0.001 per nucleotide) [7–9]. However, Mcp-oligos are inherently a complex pool of crude synthetic products containing very small quantities (10^4–10^6 molecules for each oligo) of hundreds to thousands of oligos with various errors (0.2–1 %) [9–15]. Fortunately, the problems of small oligo quantities and complex oligo pool composition can be partially resolved via high-fidelity polymerase chain reaction (PCR) amplification and the separation of the Mcp-oligo pool into subpools flanked by primers of the synthesized oligos [7, 10]. Consequently, the oligo quality becomes the primary limitation of de novo gene synthesis using Mcp-oligos.

Randall A. Hughes (ed.), *Synthetic DNA: Methods and Protocols*, Methods in Molecular Biology, vol. 1472, DOI 10.1007/978-1-4939-6343-0_17, © Springer Science+Business Media New York 2017

Here, we describe an error-removal method using an immobilized cellulose column containing a combination of two homologs of the mismatch binding protein MutS (MutS from *Escherichia coli* and *Thermus aquaticus*) to generate high-quality DNA from Mcp-oligos. After the Mcp-oligos are amplified and separated into several subpools, they are re-annealed to display the errors in the synthesized oligos as mismatches of heteroduplexes. These mismatches are then bound by a MutS immobilized cellulose column (MICC). The remaining error-depleted oligos are amplified and assembled to the target DNA segments (Fig. 1). Our protocol for error removal can be easily applied to the low-cost and high-fidelity gene synthesis using widely available Mcp-oligos with high error rates (10–30 errors/kb). Additionally, this method can be used to remove errors in DNA synthesis by traditional methods.

2 Materials

Prepare all solutions with ultrapure water and analytical grade reagents. Store all reagents at appropriate conditions.

2.1 Mcp-Oligo Subpool Preparation (See Note 1)

1. Mcp-oligos pool.
2. KOD plus DNA polymerase.
3. Standard materials and reagents for agarose gel electrophoresis.
4. UNIQ-10 oligonucleotide cleanup kit or similar.

2.2 DNA Re-annealing

1. 1 M Tris–HCl, pH 7.6: Add 80 ml of water to a 250 ml glass beaker. Weight and transfer 12.1 g Tris to the beaker and stir to dissolve. Adjust pH with 36–38 % HCl. Bring the final volume to 100 ml with water and transfer to a reagent bottle.
2. 5 M NaCl: Add 60 ml of water to a 250 ml glass breaker. Weight and transfer 29.2 g NaCl and stir to dissolve. Bring the final volume to 100 ml with water and transfer to a reagent bottle.
3. 10× Annealing buffer: 100 mM Tris–HCl, pH 7.6, 500 mM NaCl, 10 mM EDTA. Combine 10 ml 1 M Tris–Cl, pH 7.6, 10 ml 5 M NaCl, and 30 ml of water in a 250 ml glass beaker. Weight and transfer 0.372 g $Na_2EDTA \cdot 2H_2O$ to the beaker and stir to dissolve. Bring the final volume to 100 ml with water and transfer to a reagent bottle.

2.3 MutS Fusion Protein Preparation

1. Luria-Bertani (LB) broth: Add 800 ml of water to a 1 L glass breaker. Weight and transfer 10 g Bacto tryptone, 5 g Bacto yeast extract and 10 g NaCl to the beaker and stir to dissolve. Bring the final volume to 1 L with water and sterilize by autoclaving.
2. 100 mg/ml Ampicillin stock solution: Add 8 ml of water to a 25 ml glass breaker. Weight and transfer 1 g ampicillin to the

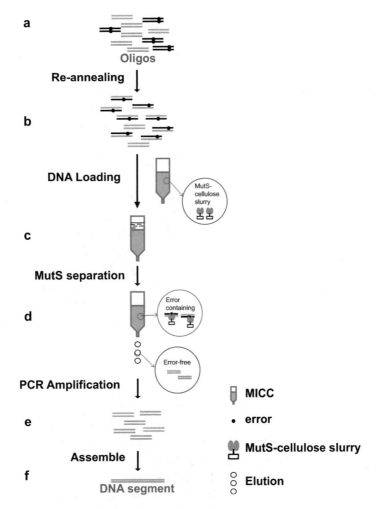

Fig. 1 Schematic representation of the MICC error-removal method. (**a–b**) Microchip-synthesized oligos are amplified via PCR and then re-annealed to expose synthetic errors as mismatches. (**b–d**) Errors are removed from re-annealed oligos using a MICC. In this process, the error-containing oligos are retained on the column and the error-free oligos pass through the column and are collected. (**d–f**) The collected error-depleted oligos are amplified via PCR and then assembled to the target DNA segments

beaker and stir to dissolve. Bring the final volume to 10 ml with water and filter sterilize. Dispense 1 ml aliquots into sterile 1.5 ml Eppendorf tubes. Store at –20 °C. Use at 100 μg/ml final concentration within 1 month.

3. 1 M Isopropyl β-D-Thiogalactoside (IPTG) stock solution: Add 8 ml of water to a 25 ml glass breaker. Weight and transfer 2.38 g IPTG to the beaker and stir to dissolve. Bring the final volume to 10 ml with water and filter sterilize. Dispense 1 ml aliquots into sterile 1.5 ml Eppendorf tubes. Store at –20 °C. Use at 1 mM final concentration within 1 month.

4. 1 M DL-Dithiothreitol (DTT) stock solution: Add 8 ml of water to a 25 ml glass breaker. Weight and transfer 1.54 g DTT to the beaker and stir to dissolve. Bring the final volume to 10 ml with water and filter sterilize. Dispense 1 ml aliquots into sterile 1.5 ml Eppendorf tubes. Store at −20 °C. Use at 1 mM final concentration within 1 month.

5. 2.5 M KCl: Add 80 ml of water to a 250 ml glass breaker. Weight and transfer 18.6 g KCl to the beaker and stir to dissolve. Bring the final volume to 100 ml with water. Transfer to a reagent bottle.

6. 2 M $MgCl_2$: Add 50 ml of water to a 250 ml glass breaker. Weight and transfer 40.6 g $MgCl_2 \cdot 6H_2O$ to the beaker and stir to dissolve. Bring the final volume to 100 ml with water and transfer to a reagent bottle.

7. Lysis-equilibration buffer (LE buffer): 20 mM Tris–HCl, pH 7.6, 300 mM KCl. Combine 2 ml 1 M Tris–HCl, pH 7.6, 12 ml 2.5 M KCl, and 60 ml of water in a 250 ml glass beaker. Bring the final volume to 100 ml with water and transfer to a reagent bottle.

8. Elution buffer: 20 mM Tris–HCl, pH 7.6, 300 mM KCl, 250 mM imidazole. Combine 2 ml of 1 M Tris–HCl, pH 7.6, 12 ml of 2.5 M KCl, and 60 ml of water in a 250 ml glass beaker. Add 1.7 g imidazole and stir to dissolve. Bring the final volume to 100 ml with water and transfer to a reagent bottle and store in the dark.

9. Wash buffer I: 20 mM Tris–HCl, pH 7.6, 300 mM KCl, 10 mM imidazole. Combine 96 ml LE buffer and 4 ml elution buffer in a 250 ml glass beaker. Transfer to a reagent bottle and store in the dark.

10. Wash buffer II: 20 mM Tris–HCl, pH 7.6, 300 mM KCl, 40 mM imidazole. Combine 84 ml LE buffer with 16 ml Elution buffer in a 250 ml glass beaker. Transfer to a reagent bottle and store in the dark.

11. Binding buffer: 20 mM Tris–HCl, pH 7.6, 100 mM KCl, 5 mM $MgCl_2$. Combine 20 ml 1 M Tris–HCl, pH 7.6, 40 ml 2.5 M KCl, and 2.5 ml 2 M MgCl in a 1 L glass beaker. Bring the final volume to 1 L with water. Transfer to a reagent bottle and autoclave. After the solution cools to room temperature, add 1 ml 1 M DTT. Store at 4 °C.

12. Dialysis membrane: Regenerated cellulose (RC), 25 KD, 8 mm width.

13. Bradford Protein Assay Kit.

14. Standard materials and reagents for sodium dodecyl sulfate (SDS)-polyacrylamide gel electrophoresis.

2.4 Regenerated Amorphous Cellulose (RAC) Slurry Preparation

1. 85 % H_3PO_4, analytical grade.

2. 2 M Na_2CO_3: Add 50 ml of water to a 250 ml glass breaker. Weight 21.2 g Na_2CO_3 and transfer to the beaker and stir to dissolve. Bring the final volume to 100 ml with water and transfer to a reagent bottle.

3. Microcrystalline cellulose (FMC PH-105,FMC Corporation, USA).

2.5 Error-Depleted Oligo Subpool Preparation

1. KOD plus DNA polymerase.

2. Standard materials and reagents for agarose gel electrophoresis.

3. UNIQ-10 oligonucleotide cleanup kit or similar.

2.6 Error-Depleted Oligo Subpool Primer Removal

1. Restriction enzyme *Mly* I.

2. Standard materials and reagents for agarose gel electrophoresis.

3. UNIQ-10 oligonucleotide cleanup kit or similar.

2.7 Oligo Subpool Assembly Components

1. KOD plus DNA polymerase, Pfu DNA polymerase.

2. Standard materials and reagents for agarose gel electrophoresis.

3. Gel extraction kit.

---

3 Methods

In this protocol, we use the de novo gene synthesis of soluble methane monooxygenase G fragment 2 (sMMO F2) [16] as an example to describe our MICC error removal and DNA assembly method.

3.1 Preparation of Mcp-Oligo Subpool

3.1.1 Design and Synthesis of the Mcp-Oligo Pool

1. All oligos for target genes are designed using the DNAWorks program (http://helixweb.nih.gov/dnaworks/) according to the program instructions [17].

2. The designed oligos are separately amplified and divided into subpools by adding different 15 bp primers, which contain *Mly* I restriction sites at each end. Each subpool contains ~10 distinct oligos, which can be used to assemble a ~350 bp DNA segment (Fig. 2).

3.1.2 Mcp-Oligo Subpool Amplification

After oligos are synthesized on the microchip, they are cleaved from the microchip by ammonium hydroxide and form a complex mixture containing all of the oligos necessary to assemble multiple genes. To simplify the assembly of these oligos into the target DNA segments, the oligo pools can be separately amplified to form different subpools by using a common flanking primer pair at each of the oligo terminals. All of the oligos in each subpool can then be assembled into the corresponding DNA segment.

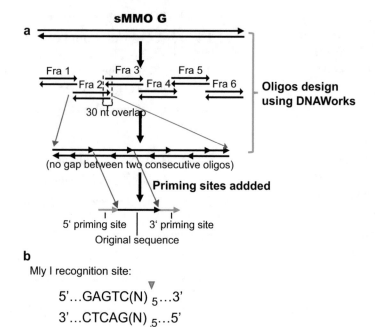

Fig. 2 Design of the oligonucleotides for de novo gene synthesis using Mcp-oligos (sMMO G oligonucleotides are described as an example). (**a**) Oligo design. (**b**) Priming site added for subpool separation

1. The oligo mix cleaved from the microchip is directly used as template for oligo subpool amplification. Each subpool is amplified by PCR with the corresponding primer pair using KOD plus DNA polymerase according to the manufacturer's instructions.

   Reaction conditions:

Primers (100 μM)	0.5 μl/each
Template (~1 ng/μl)	0.5 μl
Buffer (10×)	5 μl
dNTPs (2 mM)	5 μl
MgSO₄ (25 mM)	2 μl
DNA polymerase (2.5 U/μl)	1 μl
Water	Up to 50 μl

Cycle conditions:

1. Denaturation	94 °C	5 min	
2. Denaturation	94 °C	15 s	
3. Primers annealing	45 °C	30 s	
4. Extension	68 °C	30 s	30 cycles
5. Final extension	68 °C	10 min	

2. Load 2 μl of the PCR product on a 6 % polyacrylamide gel for analysis by gel electrophoresis (Fig. 3).

3. The remaining 48 μl of the amplified product is purified using an oligonucleotide cleanup kit according to the manufacturer's instructions. The purified oligos are eluted from the column with 40 μl of water (~100 ng/μl).

3.1.3 Re-annealing The Subpool PCR Products

The amplified subpool contains the oligos for the target gene with some oligos containing various errors. Through denaturation and re-annealing, oligos containing these synthetic errors form mismatches between the oligos with different errors or error-containing oligos and error-free oligos. The annealing products between error free oligos can still keep perfect match.

1. Combine 6 μl of 10× annealing buffer and 3 μg of purified subpool DNA in a 0.2 ml PCR tube. Bring the final volume to 60 μl with water.

2. Place the tube in a PCR thermocycler, and set the cycle condition as follows to allow the re-annealing of the PCR product (*see* **Note 2**).

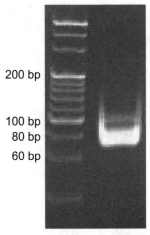

200 bp

100 bp
80 bp
60 bp

M   sMMO F2 subpool

Fig. 3 Amplification of sMMO F2 subpool. *M*: 20 bp DNA ladder marker (TaKaRa)

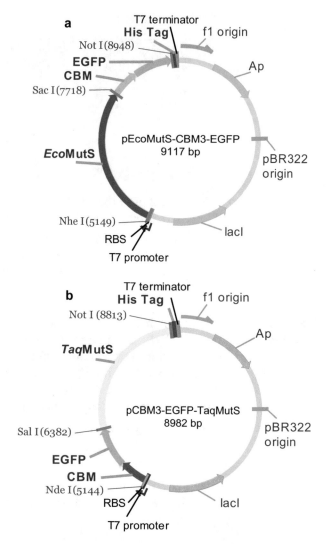

Fig. 4 Circular diagram of the expression vectors of the MutS fusion proteins. (**a**) pEcoMutS-CBM3-EGFP (eMutS expression vector). (**b**) pCBM3-EGFP-TaqMutS (tMutS expression vector)

Cycle conditions:

1. Denaturation	95 °C	5 min	
2. Re-annealing	95 °C	20 s	
	–0.1 °C/cycles	30 s	699 cycles

3.2   Preparation of MutS Fusion Protein

3.2.1   Expression of the MutS Fusion Protein

The MutS fusion protein expression plasmids were constructed in pET-21c vector (Fig. 4) [16]. The expression plasmids were transformed into *E. coli* BL21 Star (DE3) separately (*see* **Note 3**). Expression of the target gene is induced by the addition of 1 mM IPTG (final concentration) to a growing culture. Both MutS fusion proteins contain EGFP, so the protein purification can be monitored by EGFP fluorescence.

1. Pick a single colony from a freshly streaked plate and use to inoculate 3 ml of LB containing 100 µg/ml ampicillin. Incubate at 37 °C with shaking at 250 rpm overnight.

2. Use 2 ml of the overnight culture to inoculate 200 ml of LB medium containing 100 µg/ml ampicillin in a 1 L conical flask. Shake the culture at 37 °C until the OD_{600} is approximately 0.6 (e.g., 2–3 h in LB broth).

3. Add 200 µl of 1 M IPTG to the culture. Incubate the culture with shaking at the desired temperature for the appropriate amount of time (*see* **Note 4**).

4. Harvest cells in a 50 ml tube by centrifugation at $5000 \times g$ for 10 min at 4 °C. Discard the supernatant. Let the pellet drain by inversion and tap the excess medium onto a paper towel. Store at −80 °C. Use within 2 months.

3.2.2 Purification of the MutS Fusion Protein

The MutS fusion proteins contain a polyhistidine-tag at the C-terminus and can be purified using a Ni-NTA affinity column (*see* **Notes 5** and **6**). Carry out all procedures on ice unless otherwise specified.

1. Resuspend the cell pellet (generated in step 4 of the previous section) thoroughly in 20 ml of LE buffer.

2. Collect the cells by centrifugation at 4 °C for 10 min at $5000 \times g$. Discard the supernatant.

3. Thoroughly resuspend the pellet in 20 ml of ice-cold LE buffer.

4. Lyse the cells by sonication of the resuspended cell pellet using 180 one-second bursts at 30 % intensity with a 5 s cooling period.

5. Transfer the lysate to 2 ml Eppendorf tubes, centrifuge at 4 °C for 5 min at $12{,}000 \times g$ to pellet the cellular debris. Collect the supernatant in a 50 ml tube.

6. Ni-NTA column preparation: Mix the Ni-NTA slurry by gently inverting the bottle several times to completely suspend the resin. Transfer 1 ml of Ni-NTA resin slurry to a 3 ml chromatographic column. Allow the resin to settle and the storage buffer to be drained from the column.

7. Equilibrate the column with 5 ml of LE buffer.

8. Apply the cleared supernatant to the column at a flow rate of 1 ml/min.

9. After the supernatant has completely flowed through the column, wash the column with 5 ml of LE buffer.

10. After the LE buffer has completely flowed through the column, wash the column with 2.5 ml of wash buffer I.

11. After wash buffer I has completely flowed through the column, wash the column with 2.5 ml of wash buffer II.

12. After wash buffer II has completely flowed through the column, elute the MutS protein by adding 10–12 ml of elution buffer. Collect the first 8–10 ml of the elution.

3.2.3 Dialysis of the MutS Fusion Protein

1. Dialyze the MutS fusion proteins using the binding buffer at 4 °C.

2. After dialysis, transfer the target protein to 2 ml centrifugal tubes. Centrifuge at 4 °C for 5 min at $12,000 \times g$. Collect the supernatant in a 50 ml centrifugal tube. Store at 4 °C. Use within 24 h.

3. Determine the protein concentration by using 2 μl of the purified protein using a Bradford Protein Assay Kit according to the manufacturer's protocol.

4. The purified eMutS and tMutS proteins can be further verified via 4.8 % sodium dodecyl sulfate-polyacrylamide gel electrophoresis (SDS-PAGE) followed by Coomassie Brilliant Blue R-250 staining. The expected size of eMutS is 147.8 kDa, and the expected size of tMutS is 140.3 kDa (*see* **Note 7**).

3.2.4 Functional Evaluation of the MutS Fusion Proteins

The binding ability and properties of MutS to DNA are confirmed by gel shift assay (*see* **Note 8**). Four test oligos (O1, O2, O3, O4) obtained from commercial oligonucleotide suppliers (Fig. 5) can be used for this assay. Oligos O1 and O2 form 59 bp duplex with an unpaired T, and O3 and O4 form 54 bp perfectly matched duplex through the annealing of two oligos (*see* Fig. 5 and **Note 9**). According to previous studies, the mismatches corresponding to deletion or insertion errors are preferred by both EcoMutS and TaqMutS [18, 19]. Therefore, the binding of MutS to DNA containing an unpaired T and a perfectly matched DNA is used to evaluate the binding function of the MutS fusion proteins. After MutS binds to DNA, the reaction is analyzed by gel shift. The brighter smear of the free DNA in the gel represents the binding properties of the MutS fusion proteins to the duplex DNA, as the MutS–DNA complex has low mobility on the gel. A brighter smear of free DNA indicates that less DNA is bound, demonstrating a weaker binding of the MutS protein to the DNA. If the MutS fusion proteins are actively binding regions containing errors, the unpaired T DNA will be less visible if the DNA is perfectly matched. In most cases, the band of unpaired T cannot be observed (Fig. 5).

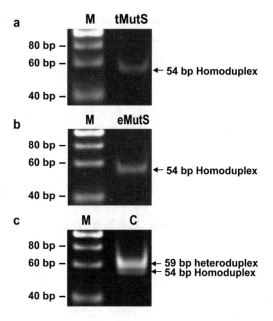

d 59 bp Unpaired T (+T)

5'–GCGGACTATTTAACACAGCTTTAGGCGCTG ACGAGGTACTATGAATCGGCCTTGCTCC–3' O1
3'–CGCCTGATAAATTGTGTCGAAATCCGCGACTTGCTCCATGATACTTAGCCGGAACGAGG–5' O2

54 bp Homoduplex

5'–GCGGACTATTTAACACAGCTTTAGGCGCGAGGTACTATGAATCGGCCTTGCTCC–3'   O3
3'–CGCCTGATAAATTGTGTCGAAATCCGCGCTCCATGATACTTAGCCGGAACGAGG–5'   O4

Fig. 5 The gel shift assay of tMutS (**a**), eMutS (**b**), and without MutS (**c**, as control) with the double-stranded oligonucleotide mixture. The 59 bp heteroduplex contains a "T" mismatch and the 54 bp homoduplex contains no errors (**d**). The DNA-MutS reactions are indicated in **step 1** of this section

1. Prepare a 10 µl reaction as follows:
   DNA-MutS reaction: 10 µl

	eMutS (µl)	tMutS (µl)	Control (µl)
59 bp Unpaired T (1 µM)	1	1	1
54 bp Perfect match (1 µM)	1	1	1
MutS fusion protein (4.0 µM)	2.5	2.5	0
1× Binding buffer	5.5	5.5	8

   Mix and incubate for 10 min at room temperature.

2. Add 3 µl of 50% glycerol to each reaction, mix, and briefly centrifuge.

3. Load 10 µl of each mixture on a 6% polyacrylamide gel (6% (w/v) acrylamide, 19:1 acrylamide:bisacrylamide, 10 mM $MgCl_2$, and 1× TBE Buffer). Run the gel at room temperature for approximately 15 min.

4. Visualize the gel by ethidium bromide (EB) staining. Scan the gel using a Gel Imaging System (Fig. 5).

3.3 Preparation of the RAC Slurry

The RAC slurry is prepared according to the method described by Hong et al. [20].

1. Add 0.2 g of microcrystalline cellulose (FMC PH-105) to a 50 mL centrifuge tube and then add 0.6 mL distilled water to wet the cellulose powder and develop cellulose-suspended slurry.

2. Slowly add 10 mL of ice-cold 86% H_3PO_4 to the slurry with vigorous stirring. Let the solution stand for 1 h on ice with occasional stirring.

3. Add 40 mL of ice-cold water at a rate of approximately 5 mL per addition with vigorous stirring between additions, resulting in a whitish, cloudy precipitate.

4. Centrifuge the precipitated cellulose at $3000 \times g$ for 10 min at 4 °C, using a swing-bucket rotor to remove the supernatant containing phosphoric acid.

5. Resuspend the pellet in ice-cold water and then centrifuge at $3000 \times g$ for 10 min at 4 °C, using a swing-bucket rotor to remove the supernatant containing phosphoric acid again.

6. Repeat **step 5** four times.

7. Resuspend the cellulose pellet with 0.5 mL of 2 M Na_2CO_3 and 45 mL of ice-cold distilled water.

8. Centrifuge the solution at $3000 \times g$ for 10 min at 4 °C, using a swing-bucket rotor. Resuspend the pellet in distilled water.

9. Repeat **step 8** once or until the solution reaches pH 5–7.

10. Store the RAC slurry as a 10 g RAC/L suspension solution at 4 °C.

3.4 Preparation of MICC

3.4.1 Pretreatment of RAC Slurry

1. Transfer 20 ml of cellulose slurry to a 50 ml chromatographic column. Allow the resin to settle and the storage buffer to drain from the column.

2. Wash the resin using 100 ml of the binding buffer.

3. After the wash buffer has completely flowed through the column, resuspend the RAC slurry with 20 ml of binding buffer. Transfer the RAC slurry to a 50 ml centrifuge tube.

4. Incubate the cellulose slurry in a 95 °C water bath for 10 min.

3.4.2 Packing of MICC

1. Mix 1 ml of RAC slurry (20 mg/ml), 600 pmol eMutS, and 600 pmol tMutS in a 1.5 ml Eppendorf tube (*see* **Note 10**). Incubate at room temperature for 10 min to allow the immobilization of the MutS on the cellulose slurry.

2. Load the MutS immobilized cellulose slurry on a chromatographic column (diameter × length: 0.4 cm × 7 cm) and drain the storage buffer from the column (*see* **Note 11**).

3. Add 1 volume of binding buffer to wash away the unbound protein. Allow the resin to settle and the binding buffer to drain from the column.

4 Error Correction by MICC

1. Mix 60 μl of the re-annealed subpool with 240 μl binding buffer.

2. Load the subpool mixture on the MICC (*see* **Note 12**). Collect the filtrates in 1.5 ml Eppendorf tubes (80 μl/tube).

3. After the supernatant has completely flowed through the column, elute with 1.5 ml of binding buffer. Collect the filtrates using 1.5 ml Eppendorf tubes (80 μl/tube).

4. Analyze 8 μl of each filtrate by gel electrophoresis using a 6% polyacrylamide gel; visualize by EB staining (Fig. 6).

4.1 Preparation of the Error-Depleted Oligo Subpool

4.1.1 PCR Amplification of the Error-Depleted Oligo Subpool

1. The chosen filtrates are used as the template for the special amplification of the oligo subpool using the corresponding primer pair. Reaction conditions:

Primers (100 μM)	0.5 μl/each
Template	0.5 μl
Buffer (10×)	5 μl
dNTPs (10 mM)	1 μl
$MgSO_4$ (25 mM)	2 μl
KOD plus DNA polymerase (2.5 U/μl)	1 μl
Water	up to 50 μ

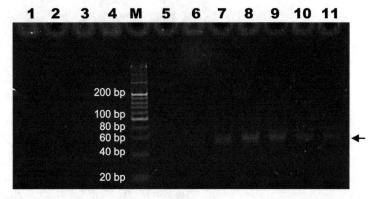

Fig. 6 Collected filtrates for sMMO G F2 subpool. *M*: 20 bp DNA ladder marker (TaKaRa Bio). *1–11*: Filtrates 1–11. The *arrow* indicates the target oligo subpool. The first several filtrates show the expected bands was used as templates for the amplification of error-depleted oligo subpool

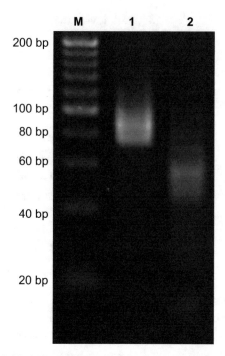

Fig. 7 The amplification and *Mly* I digestion of the oligonucleotide subpool for sMMO G fragment 2. *M*: 20 bp DNA ladder marker (TARAKA). *1*: error-depleted oligo subpool. *2*: *Mly* I-digested oligo subpool. The *arrow* indicates the cleaved 15 bp priming sites

Cycle conditions:

1. Denaturation	94 °C	5 min	
2. Denaturation	94 °C	15 s	
3. Primers annealing	45 °C	30 s	
4. Extension	68 °C	30 s	
			30 cycles
5. Final extension	68 °C	10 min	

2. Load 2 μl of the PCR product on a 6 % polyacrylamide gel for analysis by gel electrophoresis (Fig. 7).

3. The remaining 48 μl of the PCR product is purified using an oligonucleotide cleanup kit according to the manufacturer's instructions. The PCR product is eluted from the column with 40 μl of water (~100 ng/μl).

4.1.2 Primer Removal from the Error-Depleted Oligo Subpool

The primer ends of each oligos are removed by *Mly* I digestion.

1. The PCR products of the Mcp-oligos are digested using *Mly* I as follows:
   Reaction:

10× reaction buffer	10 μl
PCR products	5 μg
Mly I (10 U/μl)	5 μl
Water	Up to 100 μl

Incubate the reaction at 37 °C for 5 h.

2. Load 2 μl of the product on a 6 % polyacrylamide gel for analysis by gel electrophoresis (Fig. 7).

3. The product is purified using an oligonucleotide cleanup kit according to the manufacturer's instructions. The DNA is eluted from the purification columns with 30 μl of water (~50 ng/μl).

4.2 Assembly of the Oligo Subpool

After the primer region is removed from the oligonucleotide pool, PCA, LCR, or the combination of these two methods (LCR-PCA) is performed to assemble the target fragments (*see* **Notes 13 and 14**).

4.2.1 PCA Reaction

Reaction conditions:

Primer-removed PCR products (~50 ng/μl)	7.4 μl
Buffer (10×)	1 μl
dNTPs (2 mM)	1 μl
MgSO₄ (25 mM)	0.4 μl
KOD Plus DNA polymerase (2.5 U/μl)	0.2 μl
Water	Up to 50 μl

Cycle conditions:

1. Denaturation	94 °C	5 min	
2. Denaturation	94 °C	30 s	
3. Extension	68 °C	2 min	
			20 cycles
4. Final extension	68 °C	10 min	

Reaction conditions:

Primer-removed PCR products (~50 ng/μl)	8 μl
Buffer (10×)	1 μl
Taq DNA ligase (10 U/μl)	1 μl

Cycle conditions:

1. Denaturation	94 °C	5 min	
2. Denaturation	94 °C	30 s	
3. Extension	68 °C	2 min	⎫ 20 cycles
4. Final extension	68 °C	10 min	

1. The LCR reaction is performed as described above using 40 μl of product.

2. The reaction is purified using an oligonucleotide cleanup kit according to the manufacturer's instructions. The PCR product is eluted from the column with 40 μl of water.

3. The purified LCR products are used as the template DNA for the PCA reaction as described above (Subheading 4.2.1).

1. The PCA, the LCR, and LCR-PCA reaction products can be used as the template for the amplification of the fragments using Pfu DNA polymerase.

   Reaction conditions:

Primers (100 μM)	1 μl/each
Template	0.5 μl
Buffer (10×)	5 μl
dNTPs (10 mM)	1 μl
DNA polymerase (2.5 U/μl)	1 μl
Water	Up to 50 μl

Cycle conditions:

1. Denaturation	94 °C	5 min	
2. Denaturation	94 °C	30 s	
3. Primers annealing	Tm-3 °C	30 s	
4. Extension	72 °C	30 s	⎫ 30 cycles
5. Final extension	72 °C	10 min	

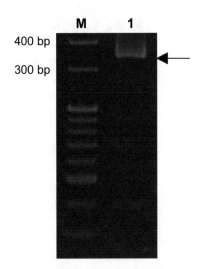

Fig. 8 sMMO G fragment 2 DNA assembled by LCR from the error-depleted oligo subpool. *M*: 20 bp DNA ladder marker (TARAKA). *1*: assembled DNA segment. *Arrow* indicates the target DNA segment (329 bp)

2. Load 5 μl of the product on a 6% polyacrylamide gel for analysis by gel electrophoresis (Fig. 8).

3. The remaining 45 μl of the PCR product is purified by gel electrophoresis using a 3% agarose gel. The target bands are cut from the gel and recovered using a gel extraction kit according to the manufacturer's instructions. The PCR product is eluted from the columns with 40 μl of water.

5   Notes

1. Other high-fidelity DNA polymerases and oligo purification kits can be used.

2. This step should take about 5–8 h. After the re-annealing, these annealed subpools should be put on ice or stored at 4 °C.

3. The MutS fusion protein expression strains are available upon request

4. For the expression of eMutS protein, incubate the culture with shaking at 16 °C for 16 h. For the expression of tMutS protein, incubate the culture with shaking at 37 °C for 4 h.

5. In many cases, the use of the affinity method enables the purification of the target protein to near homogeneity in one step. Occasionally, there are some unexpected bands of proteins after the protein purification. According to our experimental results, if the purity of the target protein is >90% homogeneous, further purification is not required.

6. Most commercial Ni-NTA affinity columns can be used to purify the fusion protein. Our purification procedure is similar to the product manual except for the use of LE buffer.

7. In most cases, the analysis of the purified proteins by SDS-PAGE can be omitted.

8. The function of the MutS fusion protein has been evaluated previously. Here, this procedure is used to confirm the activity of the fusion protein and can be used in troubleshooting. If the quality of the MutS fusion protein is good, this step can be omitted.

9. The preparation of the 59 bp unpaired T and 54 bp perfect match homoduplex is according to the procedure listed in Subheading 3.1.3 "Re-annealing of the PCR product of sub-pool"; the difference is that the final concentration of each oligo is 1 μM.

10. The molarity of MutS immobilized on the cellulose is determined based on the amount of the treated DNA sample. In our recommend protocol, the ratio of DNA sample, eMutS, and tMutS is 1:10:10, and the height of the cellulose slurry is about 2 cm. For a standard 2 cm MICC, which can be used in the error removal of 60 pmol oligos, 600 pmol eMutS and 600 pmol tMutS are immobilized on 1 ml of RAC slurry (20 mg/ml).

11. For the storage buffer to completely drain means that no additional drops of buffer will exit the column. A DNase-free column from another company can also be used.

12. The loading of the subpool must be done very carefully to avoid the spurting of the MutS-cellulose slurry.

13. In this protocol, the oligos are assembled into longer DNA fragments. However, if the aim is obtain error free oligos or error removed target DNA fragments, the assembly step is not necessary.

14. Three strategies are provided, however, if PCA or LCR only can assemble the target DNA fragment, the combination is not necessary.

Acknowledgments

This work was supported by a grant-in-aid from the National Natural Science Foundation of China (31270149), the National High Technology Research and Development Program (2012AA02A708), Anhui Provincial Natural Science Foundation (1608085MC47),the Fundamental Research Funds for the Central Universities (WK2070000059), the China Postdoctoral Science Foundation (2015M580546). This work also earned technical support from the Core Facility Center for Life Sciences, University of Science and Technology of China.

References

1. Wang HH, Isaacs FJ, Carr PA et al (2009) Programming cells by multiplex genome engineering and accelerated evolution. Nature 460:894–898

2. Carr PA, Church GM (2009) Genome engineering. Nat Biotechnol 27:1151–1162

3. Gibson DG, Benders GA, Andrews-Pfannkoch C et al (2008) Complete chemical synthesis, assembly, and cloning of a Mycoplasma genitalium genome. Science 319:1215–1220

4. Kobayashi H, Kaern M, Araki M et al (2004) Programmable cells: interfacing natural and engineered gene networks. Proc Natl Acad Sci U S A 101:8414–8419

5. Stemmer WPC, Crameri A, Ha KD et al (1995) Single-step assembly of a gene and entire plasmid from large numbers of oligodeoxyribonucleotides. Gene 164:49–53

6. Gibson DG (2009) Synthesis of DNA fragments in yeast by one-step assembly of overlapping oligonucleotides. Nucleic Acids Res 37:6984–6990

7. Kosuri S, Eroshenko N, LeProust EM et al (2010) Scalable gene synthesis by selective amplification of DNA pools from high-fidelity microchips. Nat Biotechnol 28:1295–1299

8. Gao XL, LeProust E, Zhang H et al (2001) A flexible light-directed DNA chip synthesis gated by deprotection using solution photogenerated acids. Nucleic Acids Res 29:4744–4750

9. Quan JY, Saaem I, Tang N et al (2011) Parallel on-chip gene synthesis and application to optimization of protein expression. Nat Biotechnol 29:449–452

10. Tian JD, Gong H, Sheng NJ et al (2004) Accurate multiplex gene synthesis from programmable DNA microchips. Nature 432:1050–1054

11. Richmond KE, Li MH, Rodesch MJ et al (2004) Amplification and assembly of chip-eluted DNA (AACED): a method for high-throughput gene synthesis. Nucleic Acids Res 32:5011–5018

12. Zhou X, Cai S, Hong A et al (2004) Microfluidic PicoArray synthesis of oligodeoxynucleotides and simultaneous assembling of multiple DNA sequences. Nucleic Acids Res 32:5409–5417

13. Kim C, Kaysen J, Richmond K et al (2006) Progress in gene assembly from a MAS-driven DNA microarray. Microelectron Eng 83:1613–1616

14. Cleary MA, Kilian K, Wang YQ et al (2004) Production of complex nucleic acid libraries using highly parallel in situ oligonucleotide synthesis. Nat Methods 1:241–248

15. Linshiz G, Ben Yehezkel T, Kaplan S et al (2008) Recursive construction of perfect DNA molecules from imperfect oligonucleotides. Mol Syst Biol 4:1–10

16. Wan W, Li L, Xu Q et al (2014) Error removal in microchip-synthesized DNA using immobilized MutS. Nucleic Acids Res 42, e102

17. Hoover DM, Lubkowski J (2002) DNAWorks: an automated method for designing oligonucleotides for PCR-based gene synthesis. Nucleic Acids Res 30, e43

18. Brown J, Brown T, Fox KR (2001) Affinity of mismatch-binding protein MutS for heteroduplexes containing different mismatches. Biochem J 354:627–633

19. Cho M, Chung S, Heo SD et al (2007) A simple fluorescent method for detecting mismatched DNAs using a MutS-fluorophore conjugate. Biosens Bioelectron 22:1376–1381

20. Hong J, Ye X, Wang Y et al (2008) Bioseparation of recombinant cellulose-binding module-proteins by affinity adsorption on an ultra-high-capacity cellulosic adsorbent. Anal Chim Acta 621:193–199

Chapter 18

Selection of Error-Less Synthetic Genes in Yeast

Hisashi Hoshida, Tohru Yarimizu, and Rinji Akada

Abstract

Conventional gene synthesis is usually accompanied by sequence errors, which are often deletions derived from chemically synthesized oligonucleotides. Such deletions lead to frame shifts and mostly result in premature translational terminations. Therefore, in-frame fusion of a marker gene to the downstream of a synthetic gene is an effective strategy to select for frame-shift-free synthetic genes. Functional expression of fused marker genes indicates that synthetic genes are translated without premature termination, i.e., error-less synthetic genes. A recently developed nonhomologous end joining (NHEJ)-mediated DNA cloning method in the yeast *Kluyveromyces marxianus* is suitable for the selection of frame-shift-free synthetic genes. Transformation and NHEJ-mediated in-frame joining of a synthetic gene with a selection marker gene enables colony formation of only the yeast cells containing synthetic genes without premature termination. This method increased selection frequency of error-less synthetic genes by 3- to 12-fold.

Key words In-frame fusion, *Kluyveromyces marxianus*, Nonhomologous end joining (NHEJ), Transformation, Selection marker gene, Deletion, Frame-shift

---

1 Introduction

In gene synthesis processes, chemically synthesized oligonucleotides are usually assembled by PCR to obtain long DNA fragments [1]. Therefore, accuracy of synthetic genes depends on the PCR conditions used and quality of chemically synthesized oligonucleotides. It has been shown that the PCR conditions typically used in gene assembly did not affect the accuracy of synthetic DNAs significantly [2]. On the other hand, it is suggested that up to 70% of chemically synthesized 100-mer oligonucleotides contain incorrect sequences [3]. Therefore, most of errors that occur in synthetic genes may be derived from errors in the oligonucleotides themselves. A possible way to eliminate such errors is to use high-quality oligonucleotides purified by polyacrylamide gel electrophoresis or HPLC, which reduces but does not completely remove incorrect oligonucleotides and which increases the cost of gene synthesis [1]. Another approach is enzymatic cleavage of mismatch pairs in assembled gene mixtures [4, 5]. This is applicable to

Randall A. Hughes (ed.), *Synthetic DNA: Methods and Protocols*, Methods in Molecular Biology, vol. 1472,
DOI 10.1007/978-1-4939-6343-0_18, © Springer Science+Business Media New York 2017

any sequences but requires precise adjustment of enzyme treatment condition for complete elimination of errors. The sequence analysis of a synthetic gene revealed that most of the errors observed were single nucleotide deletions which result in premature translational termination of a synthetic protein encoding sequence [2, 6]. In the case of protein-coding sequences, GFP or antibiotic resistant markers have been fused with a synthetic gene in-frame in *Escherichia coli* plasmids to eliminate such frame-shift clones and accurate gene clones were selected [6, 7]. Here we describe a simple cloning method for selecting frame-shift-free synthetic genes by using non-homologous end joining (NHEJ)-mediated plasmid construction system in the yeast *Kluyveromyces marxianus* [8].

K. marxianus has high NHEJ activity to allow joining of the ends of the DNA fragments introduced by transformation. Therefore, the NHEJ activity can be used to insert a DNA fragment into a linearized autonomously replicating plasmid [8]. This method does not require DNA end processing by restriction enzymes and ligation before transformation. A PCR-amplified DNA fragment and a PCR-amplified linear vector DNA fragment are simply mixed and directly introduced into *K. marxianus* cells, resulting in cloning of the DNA fragment in the vector through the functional marker selection system described below.

The concept to select frame-shift-free synthetic genes in *K. marxianus* is summarized in Figs. 1 and 2. This method consists of three steps, gene synthesis (Subheading 3.1, Fig. 1a), preparation of vector DNA (Subheading 3.2, Fig. 1b), and selection of frame-shift-free synthetic gene fragments through *K. marxianus* transformation (Subheading 3.3, Fig. 2). A synthetic gene is assembled from oligonucleotides by conventional assembly PCR. The resulting gene fragment pool is expected to contain inaccurate sequences. The gene fragments are amplified using primers containing flanking sequence with the 17 bp corresponding to the N-terminus of the yeast Sc*URA3* selectable marker except for the start codon ATG (Fig. 1a). The cloning vector pKM149 contains Sc*TDH3* promoter and Sc*URA3* selection marker gene, which are located in the same transcriptional direction (Fig. 1b). The vector pKM149 is amplified by PCR using the primer pair of TDH3-1c and URA3 + 21, which produces the linearized DNA containing the N-terminus-deleted Sc*URA3* (Sc*URA3ΔN*, Fig. 1b). The synthetic DNA fragments with Sc*URA3N* and the linearized vector fragments with Sc*URA3ΔN* are introduced into a *K. marxianus* ura3 deficient strain (Fig. 2). These DNA fragments are joined randomly through NHEJ. However, only when the synthetic gene lacks frame-shift deletions which result in premature translation termination, is a functional Ura3 marker protein produced. Therefore, only the yeast cells that express the synthetic gene without premature termination form colonies on the selective uracil-deficient medium (Fig. 2). The concept is somewhat

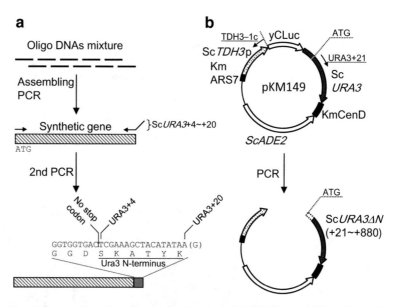

Fig. 1 Preparation of synthetic gene and vector DNA fragments. (**a**) Synthetic gene is assembled from oligonucleotides by PCR and fused with Sc*URA3* N-terminal 17 bp by a second PCR using a primer containing in-frame-designed Sc*URA3* N-terminal sequence. (**b**) The vector plasmid pKM149 consists of KmARS7; a 60 bp autonomously replicating sequence of *K. marxianus*, Sc*TDH3*p; a promoter region (−698 to −1) of *TDH3* gene of *S. cerevisiae*, yCLuc; yeast-codon-optimized CLuc (1662 bp), Sc*URA3*; *URA3* gene (−223 to +880) of *S. cerevisiae* as a transformation marker, KmCenD; a centromere sequence (248 bp) of *K. marxianus*, and Sc*ADE2*; *ADE2* gene (−797 to +1716) of *S. cerevisiae*. The vector is amplified by PCR using TDH3 − 1c and URA3 + 21 primers, resulting in the DNA fragment containing N-terminal truncated nonfunctional Sc*URA3* (+21 to +880, Sc*URA3ΔN*) and Sc*TDH3*p at each end

complex but the procedure consists of only PCR and *K. marxianus* transformation. The genetic tools for work with *K. marxianus* such as strains and plasmids are available from The National BioResource Project (NBRP) in Japan (http://yeast.lab.nig.ac.jp/nig.v2.0/index_en.html).

2   Materials

2.1   Gene Synthesis

1. Oligonucleotides are purchased from manufacturing services in 5 O.D. scale with reverse-phase cartridge purification.

2. KOD Plus DNA polymerase is used for assembly of oligonucleotides and DNA amplification in the sample synthesis of yGLuc shown herein (*see* **Note 1**).

3. PCR buffer: 10× KOD Plus buffer, 25 μM MgSO$_4$, 2 mM dNTPs. These are typically supplied together with the polymerase.

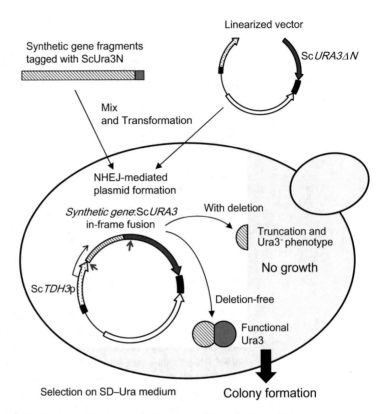

Fig. 2 Selection of frame-shift-free synthetic genes through in-frame fusion with a transformation marker. The fragments prepared as shown in Fig. 1 are used directly for the transformation of a uracil-auxotrophic *K. marxianus* mutant strain. The synthetic gene is cloned into the vector through NHEJ. In the resulting expression plasmid, the synthetic gene:Sc*URA3* in-frame fusion gene is transcribed by Sc*TDH3* promoter. If the synthetic gene has a mutation(s) causing premature translational termination, the fused Ura3 marker is not produced. On the other hand, the synthetic gene without premature termination results in translation of functional Ura3 protein. As a result, only the cells containing a frame-shift-free synthetic gene form transformant colonies on SD–Ura plates

4. 50× TAE buffer: Mix 242 g Tris base, 57.1 mL of acetic acid, and 100 mL of 0.5 M EDTA, pH 8.0, adjusted to 1 L with deionized water, and autoclaved. Dilute to 1× for agarose gel preparation and electrophoresis.

5. Agarose gel: Dissolve 1.0–1.5 % (w/v) agarose in 1× TAE buffer with 0.05 µg/mL ethidium bromide by heating with a microwave and caste in a gel tray.

6. DNA concentration measurement: Qubit® fluorometer and Quant-iT dsDNA Assay Kit (Thermo Fisher Scientific, Waltham, MA) were used according to the manufacturer's instructions. A similar spectrophotometer for DNA quantification can also be used.

2.2 Preparation of Linearized Vector DNA

1. Primers: TDH3–1c; 5′-TTTGTTTGTTTATGTGTGTTTAT TCGA-3′ and URA3+21; 5′-GGAACGTGCTGCTAC TCATCCTAGT-3′, and the PCR reagents listed in Subheading 2.1.

2. YPD: 2% Peptone, 1% yeast extract, 2% glucose, 2% agar (if necessary), autoclaved for 15 min at 121 °C.

3. SET solution: 1.2 M sorbitol, 25 mM Tris–HCl (pH 7.5), 10 mM EDTA (pH 8.0).

4. Zymo solution: Dissolve 30 mg of Zymolyase 100-T in 1 mL of SET solution containing 10% (v/v) β-mercaptoethanol and store at 4 °C.

5. 10% SDS: Dissolve 10 g of sodium dodecyl sulfate (SDS) in water and adjust to 100 mL.

6. Phenol/chloroform: A phenol:chloroform:isoamyl alcohol 25:24:1 saturated with 10 mM Tris (pH 8.0) and 1 mM EDTA reagent purchased was used.

7. RNase solution: 10 mg of DNase-free RNase was dissolved in 1 mL of water.

2.3 Selection of Frame-Shift-Free Synthetic Gene Fragments Through K. marxianus Transformation

1. SD–Ura: 0.17% Yeast nitrogen base w/o amino acid and w/o ammonium sulfate, 0.5% ammonium sulfate, 2% glucose, 0.0025% adenine hemisulfate, 0.01% L-tryptophan, 0.01% L-histidine HCl, 0.01% L-methionine, 0.02% L-leucine, 0.01% L-lysine HCl, 2% (w/v) agar, autoclaved for 15 min at 121 °C (*see* **Note 2**).

2. Transformation solution: Mix 2 mL of 60% polyethylene glycol (MW3350), 150 μL of 4 M lithium acetate, 300 μL of 1 M DL-dithiothreitol and 550 μL of water before use. One molar DL-dithiothreitol is filter-sterilized and stored at –20 °C. Stock solutions of polyethylene glycol and lithium acetate are autoclaved and stored in a refrigerator.

3. GLuc working solution: mix 1× *Gaussia* Luciferase Assay Buffer and 100× *Gaussia* Luciferase Substrate in *Gaussia* Luciferase Assay Kit (New England Biolabs, Beverly, MA) at the ratio of 100:1 before measurements.

3 Methods

3.1 Gene Synthesis

1. Design the oligonucleotides for coding sequence and reverse complementary sequence for a gene, here yGLuc [2] is synthesized (*see* **Notes 3–5**). Dissolve each synthesized oligonucleotide in water at a concentration of 10 μM.

2. Prepare a mixture containing all of the oligonucleotides to a final concentration of 0.25 μM each.

3. Make a PCR reaction mixture by mixing reagents and oligonucleotide mixture as follows: 2 μL of the oligonucleotide mixture prepared in **step 2**, 1 μL of 10× KOD Plus Buffer, 1 μL of 2 mM dNTPs, 0.4 μL of 25 mM MgSO$_4$, 0.2 μL of KOD Plus DNA polymerase, and 5.4 μL of water.

4. Run a temperature program to assemble the oligonucleotides as follows: 94 °C for 1 min, 20 cycles of 94 °C for 20 s, 55 °C for 30 s and 68 °C for 1 min/kbp. The PCR product obtained in this step is directly used in the next PCR as a template.

5. Make a PCR reaction mixture as follows: 1 μL of the PCR product obtained in **step 4**, 0.3 μL of a forward primer (yGLuc + 1, 5′-ATGGGTGTCAAGGTCTTGTT-3′), 0.3 μL of a reverse primer (URA3(+4–20)c-yGLuc + 555c, 5′-TTATATGTAGCTTTCGAGTCACCACC AGCACCCTTGA-3′), 1 μL of 10× KOD Plus Buffer, 1 μL of 2 mM dNTPs, 0.4 μL of 25 mM MgSO$_4$, 0.2 μL of KOD Plus DNA polymerase, and 5.8 μL of water.

6. Amplify the target gene fragments by the same temperature program in **step 4** but the number of cycles is changed to 30.

7. Confirm amplification of a target gene by agarose gel electrophoresis (*see* **Note 6**). The PCR solution can be used directly in the transformation step (Subheading 3.3) without further purification.

3.2 Preparation of Linearized Vector DNA

1. Inoculate a *K. marxianus* strain carrying a plasmid vector, for example pKM149 (Fig. 1), in 1.5 mL of YPD medium, and incubate at 30 °C with rotation for 18–24 h.

2. Harvest the yeast cells in a microcentrifuge tube by centrifugation, remove the supernatant with a pipette, and resuspend the precipitated cells in 300 μL of SET solution.

3. Add 20 μL of Zymo solution to the cell suspension and vortex.

4. Incubate for 30 min at 37 °C.

5. Add 200 μL of phenol/chloroform, mix vigorously, and centrifuge for 5 min at 9500×*g*. Transfer the aqueous layer to a new microcentrifuge tube

6. Add 1 μL of 10 mg/mL RNase, and incubate for 30 min at 37 °C. Then repeat **step 5**.

7. Repeat **step 5**.

8. Add 800 μL ethanol to precipitate the DNA. The DNA precipitate will appear like a tangle of thread. Discard the supernatant by decantation. Allow the DNA to dry at room temperature to remove residual ethanol.

9. After drying, dissolve the DNA in 100 μL of water (*see* **Note 7**).

10. Take an aliquot of the DNA solution and dilute it tenfold.

11. Make a PCR mixture by mixing 1 µL of the diluted DNA solution prepared in **step 10**, 0.3 µL of a forward primer (*see* **Note 8**), 0.3 µL of a reverse primer (*see* **Note 9**), 1 µL of x10 KOD Plus Buffer, 1 µL of 2 mM dNTPs, 0.4 µL of 25 mM MgSO$_4$, 0.2 µL of KOD Plus DNA polymerase, and 5.8 µL of water.

12. Amplify a linearized vector DNA by the temperature program: 94 °C for 1 min, 30 cycles of 94 °C 20 s, 55 °C for 30 s, and 68 °C for 1 min/kbp. The PCR product obtained in this step is directly used in the transformation step (Subheading 3.3) without further purification.

3.3 Selection of Frame-Shift-Free Synthetic Gene Fragments Through K. marxianus Transformation

1. To prepare transformation competent cells, culture a *K. marxianus ura3-* strain (RAK3908, [9]) in 30 mL of YPD in a 250 mL conical flask with shaking at 150 rpm for 24 h at 30 °C.

2. Harvest cells into a 50 mL tube by centrifugation at 1600×*g* for 3 min.

3. Discard the supernatant by decantation and suspend the cell pellet completely in 900 µL of the transformation solution.

4. Transfer the cell suspension to a 1.5 mL microcentrifuge tube.

5. Centrifuge the cell suspension and remove supernatant completely by a pipette.

6. Suspend the cell pellet completely in 600 µL of the fresh transformation solution. This suspension is used for transformation.

7. Dispense 50 µL each of the cell suspension into 1.5 mL tubes (*see* **Note 10**).

8. Add 100 ng each of the amplified synthetic DNA and the linearized vector DNA to a tube containing the competent cells prepared in **step 6**.

9. Mix completely and incubate at 42 °C in a water bath for 30 min (*see* **Note 11**).

10. Add 150 µL of water and mix (*see* **Note 12**).

11. Spread the cell suspension onto a SD–Ura plate. After 2–3-day incubation at 30 °C, successful colonies will appear on the plates (Fig. 3).

12. Pick several colonies produced on the SD–Ura plate and inoculate in 1 mL of YPD (*see* **Note 13**).

13. Incubate at 30 °C for 18–24 h (*see* **Note 14**).

14. If your cloned protein sequence has a functional assay compatible in cells then it maybe performed at this time to verify fully functional cloned sequences. For example, the yGluc gene synthesized and cloned as an example in this protocol could be assayed by mixing 10 µL of yeast culture with 20 µL of GLuc working solution followed by measuring the resulting lumines-

80/80 mixture   40/40 mixture

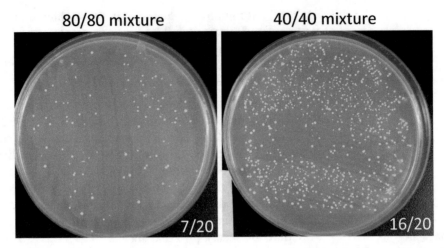

7/20   16/20

Fig. 3 Transformants generated on SD–Ura plates. yGLuc genes synthesized with 80-mer (80/80 mixture) or 40-mer (40/40 mixture) oligonucleotide mixtures were used for the transformation of a *K. marxianus ura3–* strain (RAK3908) with the linearized pKM149 vector. For selection of transformant, cells were spread on SD–Ura plates and incubated at 30 °C. The yGLuc-positive colonies/selected colonies were 7/20 and 16/20 in 80/80 and 40/40 mixtures, respectively

cence with a luminometer (*see* **Note 15**). Alternatively, the plasmid DNA could be isolated from the yeast for sequencing or further analysis in vitro.

4   Notes

1. Phusion High-Fidelity DNA polymerase has also been used for yGLuc DNA synthesis. However, any high-fidelity DNA polymerase used for PCR can be used for the frame-shift-free selection procedure.

2. As supplements stock, 0.5 g adenine hemisulfate, 2 g L-tryptophan, 2 g L-histidine HCl, 2 g L-methionine, 4 g L-leucine, and 2 g L-lysine HCl are mixed. Add 0.6 g of the supplements stock per 1 L of SD-Ura medium. The composition can be changed depending on the strains used.

3. Oligonucleotides with lengths ranging from 40 to 100 nucleotides were designed. Based on the yGLuc gene the length of the oligonucleotide did not significantly affect the efficiency of gene synthesis. The oligonucleotides must be designed to contain overlapping sequences with adjacent complementary oligonucleotides to facilitate annealing and assembly of the oligonucleotides together. The design of oligonucleotides to completely cover both strands of the desired DNA sequence enhanced synthesis efficiency in our trials. In these cases, we did not design the gene sequences to eliminate palindrome sequences, primer

dimers, or GC content of the oligonucleotides. Though these considerations may need to be considered depending on the particulars of each gene assembled from oligonucleotides.

4. Overlap sequences between adjacent complementary oligonucleotides of 20 bp generally worked well for gene assembly from oligonucleotides.

5. The Ura3 and other general yeast transformation markers are enzymes that function in the cytoplasm. Therefore, cellular localization of synthetic genes should be considered. The secretory glucoamylase from *Rhizopus oryzae* could not be directly used for in-frame Ura3 selection. On the other hand, the yGLuc synthesized with a signal sequence allowed the Ura3 marker function. Other localization signals have not been examined.

6. The PCR product in **step 4** usually shows a smear in agarose gel electrophoresis. If successful after the PCR in **step 5**, a single band corresponding to a target gene size should appear on the gel.

7. The DNA solution may be stored at −20 °C. The DNA solution contains plasmid DNA and chromosomal DNA. DNA preparation methods like colony PCR can also be used to generate the linear plasmid needed for cloning and transformation.

8. In the case of pKM149, the primer TDH3−1c was used. When other promoters are used, an oligonucleotide which anneals to the end of the promoter sequence must be designed and used instead.

9. In the case of pKM149, the primer URA3 + 21 was used. When another marker is used, a primer to amplify the marker gene sequence which deletes a nucleotide sequence encoding several amino acids must be designed to make the selection functional. In these cases, complete loss of the marker function caused by the introduced deletion should be determined before performing the selection experiment.

10. The competent cell suspension can be stored at −80 °C. Though transformation efficiency decreases gradually, competent cells can be stored for at least 6 months in our experience.

11. The transformation solution is generally highly viscous. Complete mixing must be confirmed by observing the cell suspension in the tubes while mixing to ensure that cells are distributed evenly through the mixture.

12. Mixing with SD−Ura medium increases transformation efficiency over the use of water.

13. The plasmid pKM149 is stably retained in *K. marxianus* cells even under non-selective conditions. If a SD−Ura medium is used for GLuc assay, the pH must be adjusted to around 6 with a buffer solution.

14. We generally use a 24-well plate for 1 mL of yeast culture with shaking at 150 rpm on a rotary shaker.

15. Yeast cultures were directly used for GLuc assay in this case.

References

1. Hughes RA, Miklos AE, Ellington AD (2011) Gene synthesis: methods and applications. Methods Enzymol 498:277–309. doi:10.1016/B978-0-12-385120-8.00012-7

2. Yarimizu T, Nakamura M, Hoshida H et al (2015) Screening of accurate clones for gene synthesis in yeast. J Biosci Bioeng 119:251–259. doi:10.1016/j.jbiosc.2014.08.006

3. Tian J, Ma K, Saaem I (2009) Advancing high-throughput gene synthesis technology. Mol BioSyst 5:714–722. doi:10.1039/B822268C

4. Carr PA, Park JS, Lee Y-J et al (2004) Protein-mediated error correction for de novo DNA synthesis. Nucleic Acids Res 32:e162. doi:10.1093/nar/gnh160

5. Fuhrmann M, Oertel W, Berthold P et al (2005) Removal of mismatched bases from synthetic genes by enzymatic mismatch cleavage. Nucleic Acids Res 33:1–8. doi:10.1093/nar/gni058

6. Kim H, Han H, Shin D et al (2010) A fluorescence selection method for accurate large-gene synthesis. ChemBioChem 11:2448–2452. doi:10.1002/cbic.201000368

7. Cox JC, Lape J, Sayed M et al (2007) Protein fabrication automation. Protein Sci 16:379–390. doi:10.1110/ps.062591607

8. Hoshida H, Murakami N, Suzuki A et al (2014) Non-homologous end joining-mediated functional marker selection for DNA cloning in the yeast *Kluyveromyces marxianus*. Yeast 31:29–46. doi:10.1002/yea.2993

9. Yarimizu T, Nonklang S, Nakamura J et al (2013) Identification of auxotrophic mutants of the yeast *Kluyveromyces marxianus* by non-homologous end joining-mediated integrative transformation with genes from Saccharomyces cerevisiae. Yeast 30:485–500. doi:10.1002/yea.2985

INDEX

Randall A. Hughes (ed.), *Synthetic DNA: Methods and Protocols*, Methods in Molecular Biology, vol. 1472,
DOI 10.1007/978-1-4939-6343-0, © Springer Science+Business Media New York 2017

Printed in the United States
By Bookmasters